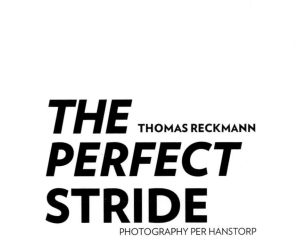

THE *THOMAS RECKMANN*
PERFECT
STRIDE
PHOTOGRAPHY PER HANSTORP

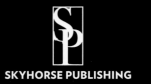

SKYHORSE PUBLISHING

THE THOMAS RECKMANN
PERFECT
STRIDE

A Runner's Guide to Healthier

Technique, Performance, and Speed

PHOTOGRAPHY PER HANSTORP

Translated by Anette Cantagallo

If you would like to get feedback on your technical training or additional tips on
how to run faster, smoother, and more efficiently, please visit
www.theperfectstride.com.

Skyhorse Publishing books may be purchased in bulk at special discounts for sales promotion, corporate gifts, fund-raising, or educational purposes. Special editions can also be created to specifications. For details, contact the Special Sales Department, Skyhorse Publishing, 307 West 36th Street, 11th Floor, New York, NY 10018 or info@skyhorsepublishing.com.
Skyhorse® and Skyhorse Publishing® are registered trademarks of Skyhorse Publishing, Inc.®, a Delaware corporation.

www.skyhorsepublishing.com

10 9 8 7 6 5 4 3 2 1

Library of Congress Cataloging-in-Publication Data is available on file.

ISBN: 978-1-62636-086-0

Printed in China

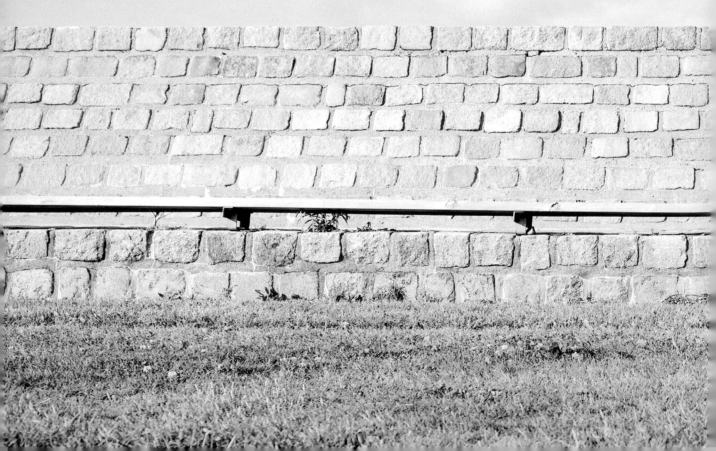

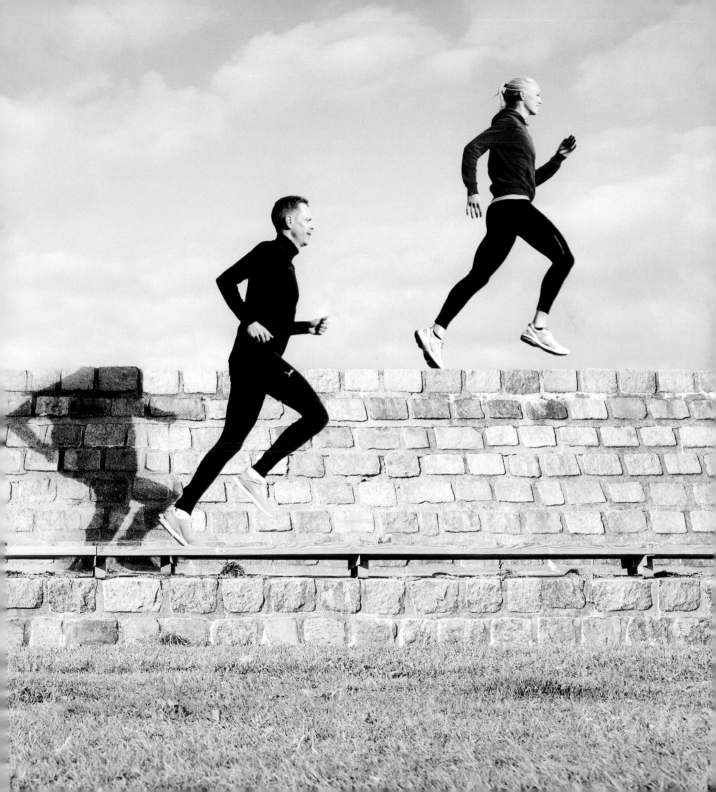

CONTENTS

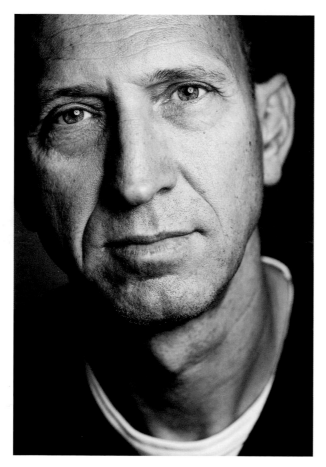

www.theperfectstride.com

THE A-HA MOMENT . . .

THE A-HA MOMENT . . .

IT HAS BEEN THREE YEARS NOW. I had just completed a crash course in yoga to do something about the tightness and back pain that usually came after running. A few days later, I ran for the first time in a few weeks. Right at the beginning, on a whim I tried to run with the body posture I learned from yoga—with elongated back, low shoulders, and a lifted chest. I thought that it would be better for my back if I ran that way instead of maintaining a high speed.

It felt like I was running without effort, and therefore I assumed I was going very slowly. After completing half of the 8 km run, I glanced at my watch. It must have shown the wrong time; given that I wasn't pushing myself, the time ought to have been several minutes later. But I let go of any thoughts about the time and re-focused on my posture. It was easier than I thought to run with my shoulders relaxed and with a more upright upper body.

At the finish line my watch showed at least five minutes faster than I had expected. The kilometer time was more than half a minute better than it ought to have been. Something wasn't right. At such a pace, I should have been exhausted by the end. Instead, I felt light and relaxed. And my back wasn't stiff or sore at all.

Slowly, it dawned on me that there was nothing wrong with the watch. The fact that the run went easily didn't necessarily mean I was running slowly. Something happened when I ran with a more upright posture—something that made the run much more efficient.

In the weeks following, I made it a point to focus on my posture. I discovered that by lowering my shoulders I ran faster without getting as tired as before. Later it became clear to me that the rapid improvement was due to the fact that I had corrected my running stride, and it immediately gave me a richer running economy—suddenly, each stride I took spent considerably less energy.

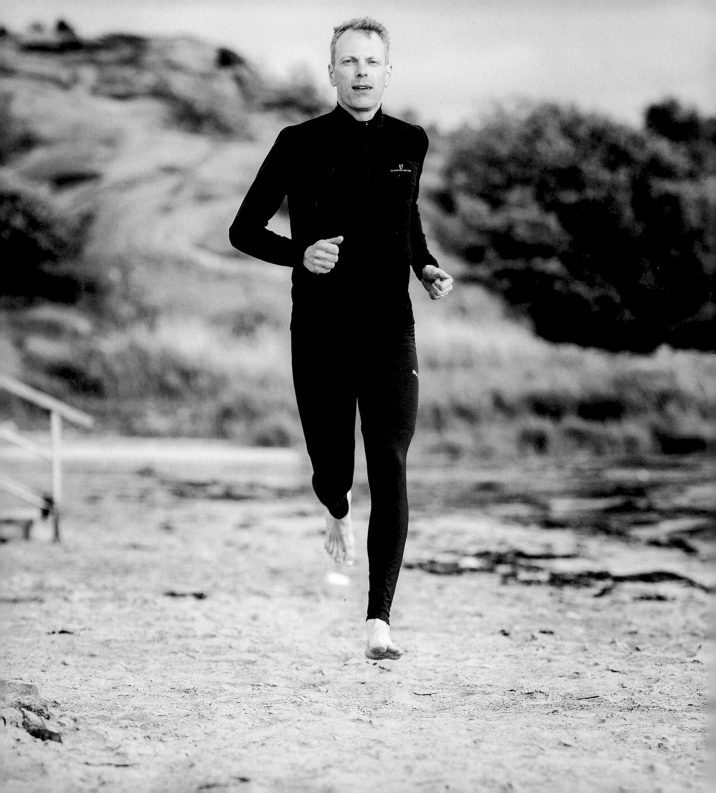

Everything starts with running technique

In recent years, a huge amount of research has shown just how important running economy is to our running capacity. When it comes to who is fastest at the elite level, the ability to run economically is more important than physical fitness. To use the analogy of a car, in long distance running it's just as important to have low fuel consumption as it is to have a large tank.

The way to a richer running economy is via a more efficient running technique, in which you take advantage of the laws of gravity instead of fighting against them. In my case, more relaxed shoulders lengthened my arm swing and gave me a more upright posture. Both factors will allow for a longer running stride without the expenditure of more energy.

To run more efficiently, you must learn to take it easy. When you want to speed up your pace or when fatigue hits you, it's relaxation that you should think of, rather than dwelling on how to push yourself harder. It may seem incongruous—we're accustomed to using maximum effort when we're performing—but when running it's more important to do it properly than to rely on maximum effort (remember to work smarter, not harder).

When it comes to running, there is a wide chasm between what the research shows and how the vast majority of us are training. Many runners are not aware that running technique decides how economic the run is and that running economy is crucial for your performance capability. This is a shame because it's not very difficult to improve your running technique.

The understanding of running needs to be updated. In sports like golf and tennis, people take lessons to improve their technique, but for running, many people believe that how they move doesn't matter. It's paradoxical, given the large enthusiasm for running. Many runners would get so much more out of their workouts—become both faster and healthier—if they just learned to run properly.

Still, there's a wide-spread belief that long distance running is only about fitness. Running magazines, books on running, and running blogs are flooded with tips on intervals, threshold workouts, and which pulse watch is the best. Few realize that it's running technique—not oxygen intake—that's the deciding factor in the African runners' dominance of the athletic track since the 1980s.

But a change may be coming. One indicator is the attention that's being paid to barefoot running, another is Christopher McDougall's international best-seller *Born to Run*, which speaks to what running is actually about—moving smoothly. Millions of people have been inspired by *Born to Run*, but what the book is missing is a description of that smooth and efficient way to run. What does it look like? And above all: How do you learn to run like that?

That was how this book was born. After reflecting on my thoughts with Johan Wettergren and Jacob Lindh, I grew convinced that there was a great need for a book for runners of all levels who wanted to learn how to run smarter. Johan is responsible for developing middle and long distance running at the Swedish athletic association SFIF and Jacob works as a sports physiologist at the Center for Health and Performance Development at Gothenburg University, where he leads an advanced project on running technique.

Shortly into the writing process, Anders Palmqvist, development manager for sprinter running at SFIF and who, like Johan, is training several elite level runners, joined the team. These three individuals have contributed their knowledge and experience and have made the book possible. Johan, who coaches at an international level in middle and long distance running, knows everything about the subject. Jacob has been invaluable for research. He has recommended a variety of surveys and examined the science in the book. Anders' role has been to convert research into practice when it comes to running economy and technology. All three have also been involved in developing the training program, which is the first of its kind.

Train holistically to become a better runner

With *The Perfect Stride*, I want to show that with only small changes to your training, you can gain a new dimension to your running and run much faster:

» Alter your training. Today, most amateur runners and many elite level runners' training programs are way too one-dimensional, focusing on their fitness at the expense of their technical training.

> **From the fifth chapter onward, there are practical exercise programs that will forever change the way you run.**

» The potential for improvement is huge. Technical training adds a new dimension, because running technique should not be limited to fitness. You'll learn how to run more efficiently and get more out of your fitness. A better running economy improves the performance ability more than several years of hard cardio training.

» It is surprisingly simple. Anyone, regardless of training background and age, can learn how to run smarter. Detect which items are crucial for your running economy and practice them.

The Perfect Stride is the first book that takes a holistic approach to running and communicates it to all ambitious amateur runners. It gives the whole picture of what running is about beyond the usual (cardio) frames, and it teaches how to run more efficiently. This is a handbook for those who want something more from running—to be faster, avoid injuries, and feel better.

In the book's practical section are numerous exercises that will make you a better runner. With a new dimension to your running, you can redesign the map of what is possible. For me, as a middle-aged runner, my new stride means that I achieve running times I have not been able to run for many years. In addition, running feels more beautiful than ever.

This book starts with theory, with a description of running economy and why running technique is so crucial to how far and fast you are able to run. In the second chapter, we look at the big picture in terms of running training: endurance, strength, and technique. After this, in chapter three, you can deepen your understanding of technical training and what is required of you for it to work. The theoretical part ends with a detailed explanation of the running stride, because, if you change your running technique, you'll need to understand what makes it more effective. From the fifth chapter onward, there are exercise programs that will forever change the way you run.

GOOD LUCK!

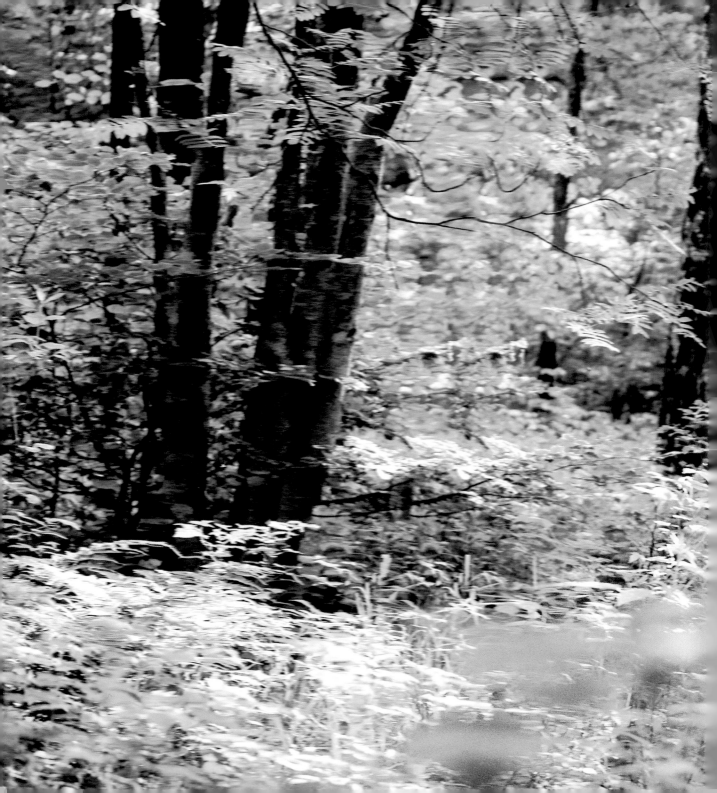

PART 1

CHAPTER 1.

FASTER, SMOOTHER, MORE EFFICIENT!

1.

INTEREST IN RUNNING HAS NEVER BEEN AS GREAT AS RIGHT NOW. Millions of people run each week and in my home country of Sweden, participation in races has increased by more than 50 percent since 2004. We run because it's healthy, to become better runners, or just to get out into nature.

Another aspect of the running boom that continues to grow is the gadget industry. Every year, Swedish runners spend around 150 million dollars on running gear. Nothing is left to chance: we buy custom shoes, functional and sweat-absorbent clothes, and compression clothing that is supposed to increase blood circulation and improve performance. Around our wrists, we strap pulse monitors and GPS watches. But maybe this is just the beginning of something even bigger . . .

For most people, running is still just cardio training, but this understanding is changing as more and more people discover what happens when they train to their entire running capacity. You don't run faster if you simply put in more effort—faster running is the result of moving correctly. Everything starts with the running stride; with a better technique, you will not only run faster, but you will reduce the risk of injury and have a much nicer running experience.

Many runners would gain so much more if they would be as particular with their training schedules as they are with their products. Shoes and other running gear, which have little effect on how fast you run, can never compensate for an inefficient running style. If you want to become a better runner then it's all about the workout, and yet there are very few runners who have embraced the available research. Therefore very few people train to their entire running capacity. Most runners practice just like they did 20–30 years ago. Or like your parents did in the 1970s— with too much emphasis on fitness.

Running is a skill that can be taught just like any other. Playing

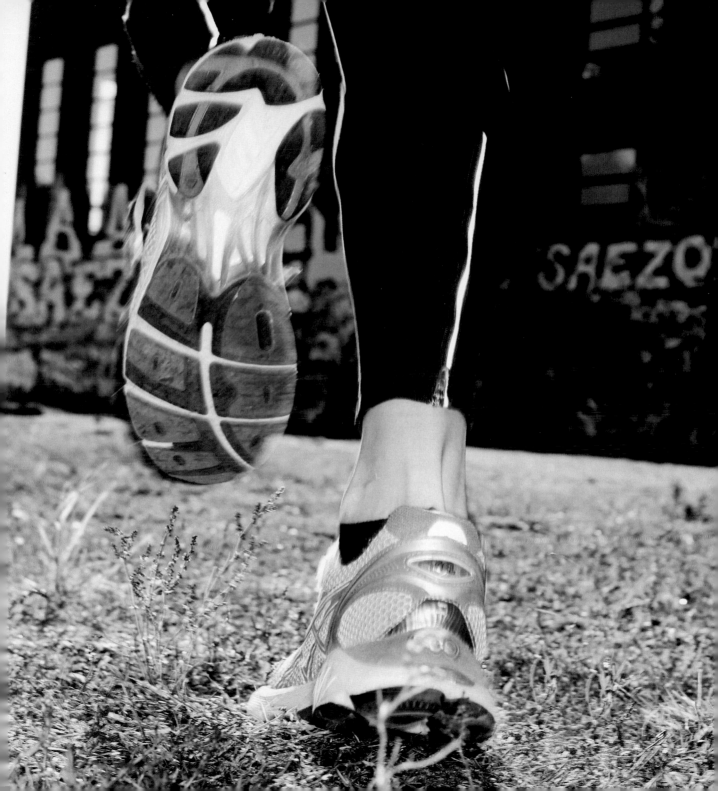

> "Even among elite level runners the ability to run energy-smart is more decisive than oxygen uptake."

tennis is much more fun if you have first learned how to hit the ball properly. It's the same with running—when you learn effective technique, the run gives you so much more. You get a completely different experience. Of course, fitness does play an important role in determining how good of a runner you are, but it only tells you about your oxygen uptake. Equally important to your capacity is how much oxygen you consume—your running economy. You cannot improve that ability by one-dimensional cardio.

Among elite level runners, the ability to run energy-efficiently is actually more decisive than fitness. Numerous studies show that Kenyan runners do not have a higher oxygen uptake (VO_2 max) than competitors from other parts of the world. They do, however, have a much better running economy, and that is where the difference lies for the East African runners—and especially those from Kenya—who have dominated long distance running since the 1980s.

Thanks to a more economical running stride, they run just as fast as other runners but with lower oxygen consumption, which is crucial for endurance. This means that Kenyan runners do not incur the same amount of lactic acid, and therefore they can maintain a higher pace for a longer time.

Running economy can vary up to 30 percent for runners with equally good fitness, and with that in mind, it is easy to understand the tremendous benefits it has for performance. This corresponds to a difference of at least 60–90 seconds in kilometer-time or 25–30 minutes in a half-marathon. At the elite level, the variation is lower, 10–15 percent. Why there is a lesser difference in that group is because everyone there already runs fairly energy-efficiently—otherwise they wouldn't be elite runners.

Running technique paves the way to speed

You can improve your running economy just like you can your fitness levels. The reason why more people are not engaging in improving their running economy is probably because they don't know just what a major role energy consumption plays and how easy it actually is to boost it. Research shows that good running economy is characterized by

» the body's center of gravity moving up and down minimally

- » the knee pointed forward when the leg swings forward

- » landing on the ground on the front part of the foot

- » the runner pushing forward instead of pulling forward

- » good flexibility in the hips

- » elastic muscles

- » upright posture

- » strong stabilizing muscles in the torso

What everything on this list has in common is that you can improve on it through practice. It is no more complicated than that. If you want to improve your running economy, then you need to practice your running technique. Your running technique is the stepping-stone, and better running economy is the goal.

The definition of technically good running is that it requires the lowest possible consumption of energy. Haile Gebrselassie, considered by many to be the best long distance runner of our time, is famous for his efficient technique and his running stride, which naturally meets all the above criteria. In this book we focus primarily on three factors: the hip work, posture, and the landing of the foot. If you learn those aspects, then you'll get the others into the bargain, but it's actually enough to improve only one of them—either the hips, posture, or the way the foot lands—to become a much better runner.

The perfect running stride is unattainable for most people, but the closer you get to Gebrselassie's way of running, the more economic running you'll be able to achieve. You lower the energy consumption and run faster.

Later, we'll return to the African runners and look at what we can learn from them in order to run more efficiently. But we can already state that running economy combined with fitness determines how fast and how far you are able to run. Physical fitness helps you maximize oxygen intake from the air inhaled, and running economy allows you to get as much as possible from the oxygen you inhale.

Running training is all about becoming as good as you can. But if you opt out of technical running and instead train cardio alone, this is about as poorly planned as a race car built with a strong engine but with no thought for the design of the body.

A car is fast not just because it has a powerful engine, but because it has a streamlined design that reduces air resistance. Running works in a similar way; even though it's gravity that has to be overcome rather than air resistance, the running stride is just as important as a strong engine (the heart).

A new dimension

Back in the 1930s, physicists discovered that different runners consumed different amounts of oxygen even though they ran at the same pace. This is the origin of research on running economy. Running economy is measured by how much oxygen a person consumes in one minute divided by body weight. In practice, this works by measuring the exhaled air of a person running on a treadmill. The less oxygen you consume at a given speed, the more energy-efficient your run will be. A common speed when studying runners' efficiency is 268 meter/minute, equivalent to a kilometer time of 3.44 minutes. At this speed the average oxygen consumption is 50.3 ml oxygen/minute/kg. The lowest measured value is 39 ml, which was found in an African runner. This is 22 percent better than average and shows how vastly running economy can vary between individuals.

> **66 The definition of good technical running is that energy consumption is the lowest possible. 99**

Although running economy is decisive, so few of the world's presumably half a billion runners train to improve it. Great care is given to the engine, but the body is forgotten. Many are practicing intervals, threshold training, fast distance, long distance, and they believe this is varied training when really they're just different variations of cardio training.

The problem with unilateral training is that the effects of the training level out much quicker, and you'll simply stop developing. Studies of elite athletes show that even after one year of intense cardio training, the oxygen uptake will only marginally improve. Running economy, however, is a quality that can, with practice, be developed for at least 6–8 years before it starts to reach a plateau. Commonly elite level runners who practice versatile training reach their fitness peak in their 20s, but by running more economically they will continue to improve their running ability for another ten years.

If you want to run with lower oxygen consumption, you must practice your running stride. Running is performed by your muscles, and they are controlled by the brain through the nervous system; therefore, it's not your physical fitness but instead your strength, flexibility, and coordination that set the limit for how efficiently you run. Technical training is about teaching your muscles to work as efficiently as possible. Running with efficient technique makes your muscles use less oxygen as it takes advantage of the laws of gravity instead of fighting against them.

Technical training adds a new dimension to your running, because you train the capacity of your nervous system, which is something that can't be achieved through cardio training. Your endurance improves because you use less energy, and this is completely independent of physical fitness. If you adjust your running style, for example, by running with a more upright posture, it reduces energy consumption considerably and therefore affects your running much more than new shoes or compression clothing ever could. As you start to run faster, you'll notice that you can also run longer without using more effort. Instead of thinking about running faster, you'll be thinking about running correctly. This way you'll go faster without consuming more energy.

The main benefits of a better running technique are that you

» become a faster runner

» prevent injuries

» increase your wellbeing,
  both physically and mentally

Take a holistic approach

A more efficient running style will help you achieve your full potential as a long distance runner. When you supplement cardio training with technical training, you obtain the additional tool of an improved endurance. You take a holistic approach to running but without having to train harder—just smarter. One plus one equals three. Technical running is also more fun and less strenuous than pure cardio training.

With a more efficient running technique your body will also be more relaxed when you run. Because a relaxed running style is more natural to the body, the risk of injury decreases. According to a much-quoted article from *British Journal of Sports Medicine* (2004), eight out of ten runners are affected by overuse injuries, and most running injuries are caused by a poor running technique that places extra stress on muscles and joints. This is why a better running technique is the foundation for better health.

But if by practicing better running technique you will become both faster and less injury-prone, why do so few actually do it? Probably this is in large part because of the power of tradition. The importance of fitness has been known ever since the emergence of the sports movement in the 1900s. However, knowledge of the brain's ability to learn new movements only gained traction in recent years. And it's easier to measure the effects of cardio training because for that all you need is a watch. Few are aware of the other side of the coin— that the effects of cardio level out faster than the improvements caused by practicing your running technique.

The reason why technical training shows results more slowly is because it trains the nervous system rather than the heart and lungs. It takes time to learn to ride a bike, but once you learn, you have the ability to ride a bike for the rest of your life.

When practicing your running technique, your focus should be on doing it correctly. If you're performing the exercises half-heartedly or improperly, you miss the learning and the training is wasted. This book's training program has been designed for you to be able to get past the most common hurdles. You must, for instance, have a muscular

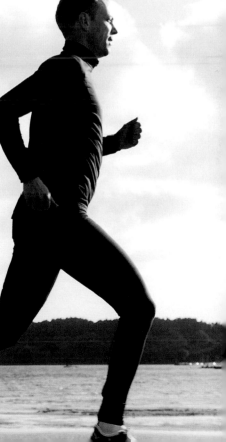

base to be able to learn a new technique, and therefore, special flexibility and strength exercises are included.

In this program you will first learn the right techniques through basic exercises and then try to bring those techniques into your running. Eventually you will get a faster stride that improves your running ability more than you could ever achieve with intense cardio training. Unlike intervals and other exercises that improve the pulse, the effect is long-term. Performing with running economy is a quality you can improve throughout life, regardless of your fitness level.

Technique is key

In sports like tennis and golf, it's logical to take classes in technique in order to improve your swing or groundstroke. Running, however, is sometimes regarded as an activity in which technique is impossible to change, or in which it doesn't matter. But why would technique be irrelevant in running?

Like golf and tennis, running builds upon some basic technical skills that are crucial for both performance ability and injury avoidance. In running, you should work actively with the hips, land on the front part of the foot, and carry yourself with an upright posture. This can be compared to tennis, where the player must have good footwork in order to get to the ball and a long stroke with which to hit the ball with power. In golf, you must begin from a good basic stance and have the right grip on the club in order to create optimal conditions for the swing.

Good technique is just as important in running as in golf and tennis, and therefore it should be as obvious for runners that they need to correct their running style as it is for golf and tennis players to work with their club or racquet techniques. It's not as though the proper movements automatically occur as soon as you start to run. Running without correct technique only leads to the consolidation of energy-inefficient strides.

> **"In this program you will first learn the right techniques through basic exercises and then try to bring those techniques into your running."**

Fortunately, it's easier to improve your technique in running than in many other sports. Firstly, the movements are much slower than when you, for instance, swing a golf club or backhand a tennis racquet, which means they are easier to control. Running is both more natural and original than the sand-trap golf swing or a tennis smash. Moreover, technical training in running is easier because unlike many ball games, you don't need to consider how your opponents might act. You can be 100 percent concentrated on what you yourself are doing—trying to run correctly.

Adding to that, the running stride is repeated several times per second, which allows you to practice a new movement many times in a short amount of time. Thus, learning occurs much faster than when practicing something like a golf swing.

These differences make sports like golf and tennis far more complex than running and therefore they may require the help of a personal trainer to improve technique. In contrast, running technique is something you can do with a good exercise program and improve on your own.

The technique behind the Swedish track and field wonder

For a long time, track and field has understood the significance of technique. With regards to coordination exercises, it's still far ahead of soccer and other team sports. All events—except the middle and long distance running—are "technical events." But the division does not mean that technique is irrelevant when you run long distance, as we have already highlighted. The only significant difference between running longer distances and other track and field events is that in longer races you also depend on your oxygen uptake.

It was advanced technical training that lay behind the Swedish athletic wonders during the first years of the 2000s. The success of Olympic champions Carolina Klüft, Christian Olsson, Stefan Holm, and other stars did not depend only on talent. They were technically also extremely well-drilled, and that is important in the jump events where technique and timing become increasingly important at the expense of physical strength.

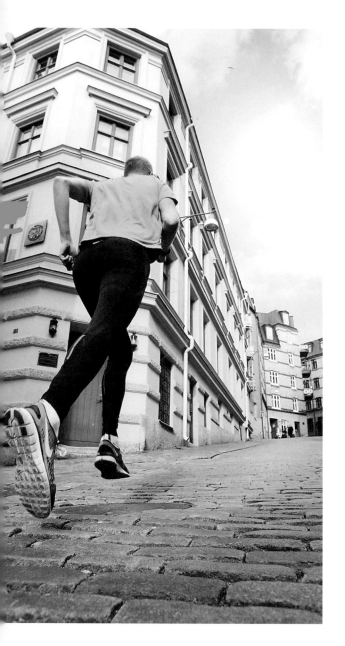

Before the World Cup final in the triple jump in 2003, a newspaper wrote that Christian Olsson was the participant who had the weakest leg strength, despite his personal best in the squat. But like in the 10,000-meter final, where the runners with efficient running techniques are the ones who win, in the triple jump it's equally important to move efficiently. It's not all about strength. Therefore, Christian became the world champion even though his competitors were more muscular.

The Swedes' skills, particularly in the jump events, depended to a large extent on the scientific knowledge several elite level coaches had picked up from Eastern countries after the fall of the Berlin Wall. Athletic research in the former Soviet Union and the GDR was far more advanced than in the Western world and was about much more than doping. Based on knowledge about the human body, science-based training techniques had been developed that helped athletes jump 2.30 meters in height or throw the discus 65 meters in length.

Sweden's coaches' technical expertise compensated for the comparatively few naturally talented athletes Sweden had. Those who were considered the most talented received the better training. What followed was the spread of that knowledge and today similar training is practiced worldwide.

The Swedish athletic wonder was limited to the so-called "technical events", such as jump and hurdle competitions. In middle and long distance running, we have been far behind Kenya and several other African nations since the 1980s.

Why do my native Swedes reach world elite levels in technical events but not in long distance running? Is it because we haven't learned to take advantage of our technical expertise when it comes to long distance running? Or is it that only in African runners understand that long distance running is also about technique . . . ?

The Kenyan running wonder

In 2011, the world's top twenty male marathon runners were from Kenya. Remarkably, the best European runner had no fewer than seventy Kenyans in front of him! On the women's side, runners from Kenya and Ethiopia were almost as superior. And the dominance was great even at shorter distances— at the men's 3,000-meter run, five Kenyans and Ethiopians were at the top, while the runners from both countries secured the first ten places at the women's 5,000 meter run.

There has been much speculation about why East African runners, especially the Kenyans, dominate so strongly. But the research is clear— the difference is in their superior running economy. The East African runners are no more physically fit than runners from the rest of the world. Thanks to more efficient running, an average Kenyan runner consumes 8 percent less oxygen than Western runners at the same speed. This is not a small difference—8 percent of the final time in a 10,000-meter run will be just over two minutes.

Where does their superior running economy come from?

It's clear that the difference isn't due to Kenyan runners' lives and training at a higher altitude because that affects only the ability to carry oxygen, not how much they consume. Another explanation for the Kenyan running miracle that can be erased is that Kenyans have to train harder for a successful running career in order to save themselves from poverty. Greater motivation can, of course, increase your willingness to make the effort, but if you push yourself too hard you actually work against your ability to run more efficiently.

No, the real reason for their dominance on the track is that East-African runners have more efficient running techniques. We have already noted that a good running economy is characterized by a number of factors, almost all of which have to do with running technique. In-depth studies of runners from countries like Kenya and Ethiopia show that, compared with European runners, they run with more pointed knees in their stride, meet the ground on the top of the foot, have a broader range of motion in the hips, and so on.

Their better running technique also depends partly on the fact that the runners from East Africa have slightly smaller and lower legs, which favors the forward stride of the leg, similar to when you switch to a lighter shoe. But the main reason is that the Kenyans run barefoot up until the age of seventeen. Without shoes, running automatically becomes more natural and effective—if you land on the front part of the foot, the body stays more upright, while the hips push the body forward, which means that the runner's bodyweight powers him or her forward. Thanks to several thousands of miles of barefoot running on gravel surfaces, the Kenyans learn to run efficiently and with the lowest possible energy consumption from the very beginning. They never have to practice their technique as they already know how to run correctly, unlike, for example, American youths who practice just as much in shoes. Shoes restrict the foot's natural movement and cause the body to become adjusted to using an inefficient technique. American runners who continue the training program learned in their youth will have already learned an incorrect stride, and therefore will not achieve the same results from their workouts. The difference lies in quality and not in quantity—it's more important to run correctly than to run long distances but, ideally, you should do both.

The large amount of barefoot running also provides much stronger feet and calves, which allows Kenyan runners to have a faster foot landing. They also gain greater elasticity in their muscles, which both reduces energy consumption and allows them to train harder than Western runners. If in the future we are to be able to compete with African runners in middle and long distance running, then the American running youth will also have to spend a large amount of time running barefoot from an early age. Unfortunately, most American and European climates don't make this easy to implement in practice. However, athletic clubs should make sure that from the beginning, the running youth should get accustomed to running in shoes with thin soles and without heel build-ups, in order to mimic the barefoot step as much as possible.

The benefits of barefoot running do not mean that you should immediately stop wearing running shoes. However, you should replace them with shoes with thinner soles, if you have not already done so. But we will come back to this later.

"The secret" behind the Kenyans' success is not any advanced training methods. It's a twist of fate that they are forced to run barefoot early in their career because of a lack of shoes, but this is what gives them an advantage in technique and strength. The most natural running stride is the most effective, and it is much more important than moderated shoes, compression clothes, and GPS watches.

Natural = Fast

Over the course of millions of years, human beings have developed a way to run that is most effective. Thanks to evolution, we carry the perfect running stride in our genes. We are born to be good runners. Just look at how children run—their posture is upright, they land with a foot under the body, and they press forward.

In *Born to Run*, Christopher McDougall describes how Mexico's Tarahumara Indians retain a natural running style into their adulthood and are therefore the world's best ultra-distance runners: "That was the real secret of the Tarahumara: they'd never forgotten what it felt like to love running. They remembered that running was mankind's first fine art, our original act of inspired creation. Way before we were scratching pictures on caves or beating rhythms on hollow trees, we were perfecting

> **66 Over the course of millions of years, human beings have developed a way to run that is most effective. 99**

the art of combining our breath and mind and muscles into fluid self-propulsion over wild terrain."

The natural, innate running stride as a whole is built on fitness, strength, and technique. When physiologists study running techniques based on gravitational force and biomechanics, they discover that the most natural way to run is also the most efficient. The Tarahumara Indians run with a foot landing similar to the one Kenyans have. The landing is under the body on the front of the foot in a quick and gentle running style that unloads knees, hips, and back.

Unfortunately, only a fraction of all runners in the Western world run naturally and efficiently, which is undeniably paradoxical given that we spend so much time and money on running. Most people run the same way as they walk, placing the heel in front of the body and wasting energy on pulling themselves forward instead of using their bodyweight to create forward force.

One reason why we have lost our innate running stride is that our modern running shoes, with their heavy soles under the heel, make running more unnatural. But the main reason why many people run stiffly and inefficiently is because we sit still for a large portion of our waking hours. Starting in kindergarten, we spend uncountable hours each day sitting in a chair, and because our bodies are built for movement, physical inactivity creates stiff muscles, poor posture, and poor flexibility.

Regular running training is not enough to prevent stiff joints as long as it focuses only on cardio. It's been said that today's running fad has saved many a heart but destroyed uncountable knees and other joints. In order to get a proper balance in the body, you must also train muscle strength, technique, and movement. This is the same practice that teaches you how to run more efficiently.

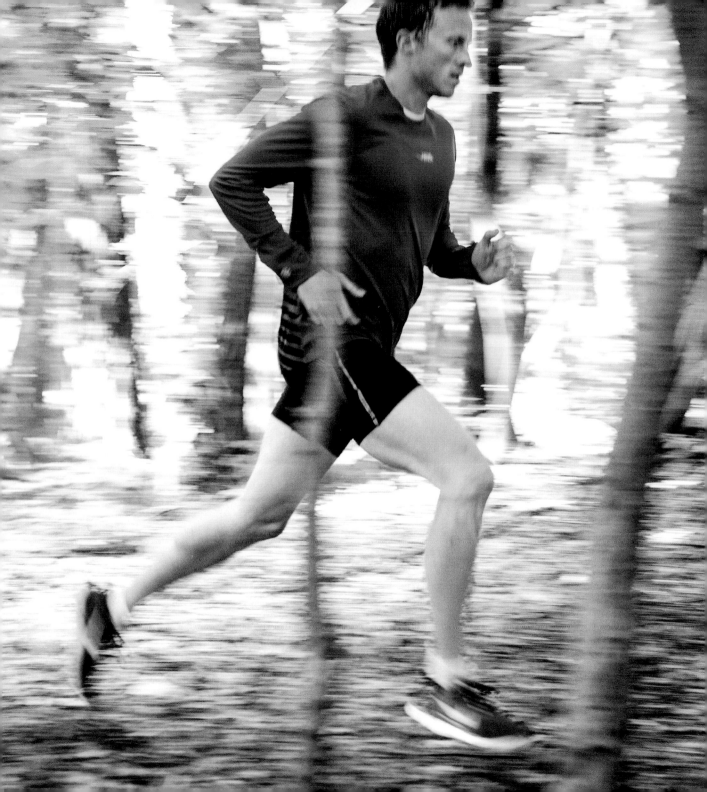

The Runner's High!

Practicing technical running involves finding your way back to that original running stride. The reward is better health in all aspects: you get greater body awareness, and flexibility in the hips and shoulders that not only makes you run faster, but also reduces the risk of injury. In addition, you will move more smoothly and relaxedly even outside the running track.

But a more natural running stride also has a psychological impact. If you've ever attained a runner's high, you know what it means for your sense of wellbeing

You end up in a state where your body just flows on by itself without any sporadic or jerking movements, and it's a pleasure to run. Running becomes an end in itself, instead of being a means to another goal, such as shedding pounds or cutting seconds.

That feeling of wellbeing is probably because we have running in our genes. Recent anthropological research has shown that running has been an important part of humanity's survival, and because of this we may feel a particularly great sense of satisfaction from running in certain circumstances. A runner's high comes when you run a long distance without having to use too much effort. This is exactly what happens when you find your way back to your natural running stride; you run with lower energy consumption and can run faster and longer without getting a buildup of lactic acid. After running at your natural stride, you feel euphoria instead of fatigue, even if you've run faster than you have in years.

When you're experiencing a runner's high, endorphins and other neurotransmitters related to euphoriants are secreted in the body. Unlike morphine, which produces a similar effect, the pleasant feeling you get from natural running alone is healthy.

Running is beneficial to your mental health even when you don't experience a runner's high. Several studies show that running is more effective than medication in combating depression. The reason for this is that a certain amount of endorphins are released in the body as soon as the heart rate reaches a high enough level. Running also reduces stress hormones. These positive effects will be much more obvious to you if you learn how to run more naturally and float through your run instead of forcing yourself forward with a stiff body.

With better technique, you get more out of your running. Smoother steps provide a greater sense of presence that takes you even further away from everyday demands: you're in the moment and enjoying every stride instead of thinking about accomplishing those kilometers. Running becomes something other than just physical training, whether you already run regularly or simply run occasionally for fun.

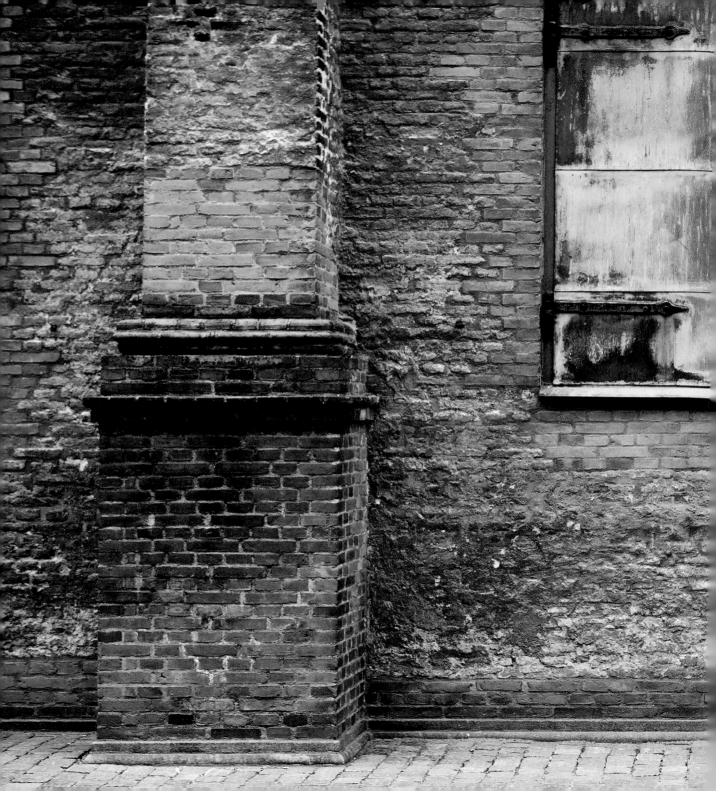

CHAPTER 2

THE FOUNDATIONS OF RUNNING

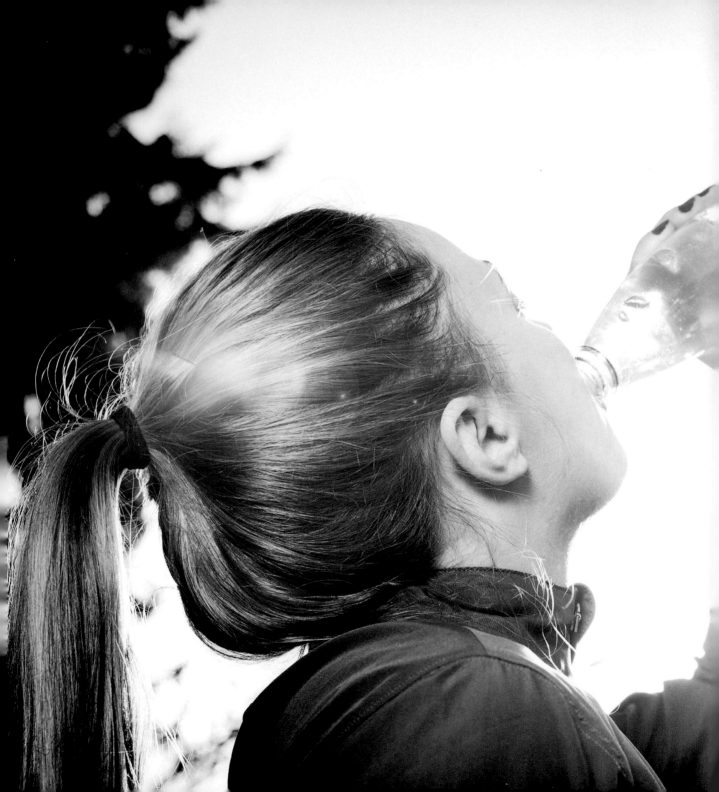

2.

ALL ATHLETIC PERFORMANCES ARE BASED ON A COMBINATION OF THREE FACTORS: fitness, strength, and technique. This applies whether you are playing soccer, wrestling, doing the high jump, long distance running, or any other physical activity.

1. Fitness releases energy

2. Muscles create strength

3. Technique saves energy and increases strength

Physiologists call the above performance factors—the three basic qualities that can improve your performance. Between different sports, there is obviously a big difference in which qualities are most important. In power sports, such as weightlifting and shot-put, it is important to develop maximum power; this is why you train muscular strength above everything else. In other sports, like the pole vault and golf, it's all about moving as technically and correctly as possible; therefore, training is focused on the interaction between the brain and the muscles, thereby teaching the muscles what to do. Although muscle strength is important in the pole vault it will still come in second—you have no use for strong muscles if you're unable to use them properly.

Long distance running falls into a third group of sports where it's important to have good physical fitness and be able to work at a relatively high intensity for a long period of time. But in running—as well as in cross-country skiing, for example—technique plays an important role in success. Even though it is possible to run a marathon with poor running technique, there's no doubt that by running more efficiently, there is a huge potential for improvement.

Fitness

When you run, your muscles do the mechanical work. But after a few minutes your muscles must be filled with new energy in order for you to be able to continue. This energy comes from the oxygen in the air you inhale. Your ability to work out for a long time is in large part determined by your physical fitness, which in turn is dependent on your heart, lungs, and blood vessels. But it's not enough to train your fitness if you are a long distance runner.

The misconception that running is just about fitness originated in the 1960s. That was when running started to be regarded as beneficial to public health, because the risks that came with more and more people having sedentary jobs were discovered. Fitness training boosts the body's metabolism and has positive effects on the heart and bodyweight. Therefore, running became something exclusive to improving one's fitness. That running could provide something more was not considered. And that notion has stuck around since then.

The obsession with cardio is the reason why most running tracks from the 1960s and '70s are so hilly. The more numerous and the steeper the slopes, the greater the effect on your fitness. If you get that far, that is. We have to wonder how many beginners get discouraged from running because of the hilly tracks that cause thighs full of heavy lactic acid after only a few minutes. The severity of the track is important for motivation, especially for moderately trained people, and this is probably one of the reasons why the much flatter city races have become so popular. On flatter land you're not forced to constantly bite the bullet to get up the tough hills.

VO₂ max tells how hard you work out

Cardio's first link is when you inhale air into the lungs. Air contains oxygen, which is taken up in the blood and transported to the muscles, where it is burned and converted into the energy that is your fuel when running. Cardio exercise improves oxygen transport. If you exercise regularly, your lungs become better at breathing in the air, the heart can pump more blood, and the muscles increase their oxygen uptake. That way, the body can access more energy, and you can work out harder. Your fitness is measured in maximum oxygen uptake (VO_2

max), or rather how many milliliters of oxygen per kilogram of body mass that your body is able to transport per minute. VO_2 max tells how hard you can manage to work out while running a race, for instance. The value is not so much about how long you manage to work out for at a fast pace. Research shows that VO_2 max has a much clearer connection with running time on the distances 800 meters and 1,500 meters than with the time for 10,000 meters or longer distances.

The most effective way to improve your fitness is via intervals. The purpose of intervals is that you can run a lot faster because the distance is shorter than a usual workout or race. The faster pace forces the entire circulatory system to work at a higher level, and the lungs, heart, and muscles are subjected to a tougher strain that increases the ability to carry oxygen.

If the intervals are to improve your fitness, then the active running sessions need to be long enough. The tougher the pace, the closer you will get to your maximum oxygen uptake and the shorter the total interval race needs to be.

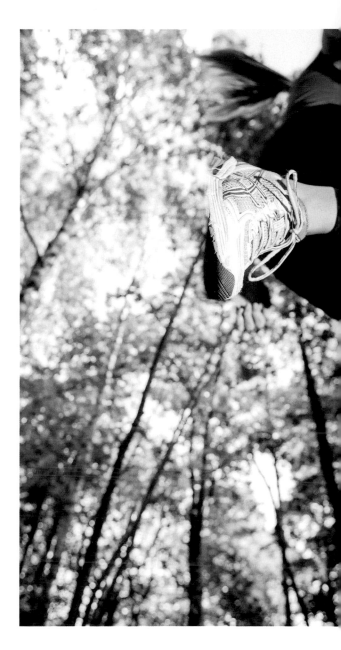

Typically at least 15–20 minutes of training is required.

When you do cardio, it's primarily the heart's stroke volume that increases. For untrained runners, the amount of blood the heart pumps out each time it constricts can increase by 40 percent within 3–4 months. Within the same time frame, physical fitness may improve up to 20 percent. After that, development continues at a slower pace, no matter how much you practice. After about a year of intensive training, it's difficult to improve your fitness any further. But luckily, endurance can continue to develop if you practice running economy.

Slow and Steady

Running long distances at a slower pace has no great effect on your maximal oxygen uptake. However, it does affect your running economy a little, as the muscles in your legs will get better at taking up oxygen from the blood for a longer period of time. We all know how important muscle endurance is—we've experienced thigh and calf pain when our energy is low during the last few kilometers of a long distance run.

To reduce the risk of suffering convulsive muscle fatigue, you can prepare for a full or half marathon by working your muscles for the same amount of time as the race will take. It does not matter if you run slower during this exercise session than your intended pace during the race. The point is that the muscle's energy metabolism is operating for long enough.

Just remember that a few hours of cycling or cross-country skiing doesn't have the same effect on the muscles used in running. Fitness training in other sports is great exercise for your general physique and for your heart and lungs, but because the movements are different, the metabolism in the muscles you use when running will not improve as much.

Another benefit of running long distances at a slower pace is that you are able to give more concentration to your running technique. You have more energy leftover to focus on posture, hip position, or any other detail of the running stride. The longer you manage to run technically correctly, the more your muscles get used to working more efficiently, and the learning effect becomes greater. But this, of course, requires that you maintain a sufficient speed so your running stride is similar to what it is at full speed. The goal is that you will later be able to run energy-efficiently when running fast.

Muscle Force

It's the muscles that create the dynamic of your running stride by shifting between engagement and relaxation. Certain muscles work during each step of the stride, while counteracting muscles, known as antagonists, are relaxed. One example is in the foot push-off: the muscles of the front thigh stretch while the hamstring muscles at the back of the thigh relax. When the leg strides forward with a pointed knee, it's the muscles at the back of the thigh that bend the leg, and the front muscles are relaxed. The process is repeated over and over again in every step.

The thigh muscles' work in the stride occurs automatically, and you don't need to think about how you're doing it. This is because the running motion is automated and controlled from a part of the brain that's outside your consciousness. When learning a new move you'll have to think about how to do it because the brain doesn't have any finished nerves for the task.

The muscles are important for your running economy, and they

> **❝ It's the muscles that create the dynamic of your running stride by shifting between engagement and relaxation. ❞**

need to develop as much force as possible to keep your body in the right position to run with technical correctness. To manage that, the muscles must be strong, flexible, and well coordinated.

Strength keeps your body in the correct position

At the landing of each stride, your body has to absorb a vertical force that is up to three times greater than your own bodyweight. To counter that power you have to be strong in the calves, thighs, buttocks, and back—the muscles that hold the body upright. Runners who are too weak in that chain collapse upon landing, and it impairs their running economy heavily because the body's center of gravity should move as little as possible vertically. Too-weak extension/stretch muscles are also the most common reason for running injuries.

In Chapter 9, you'll find a complete strength program for runners; if you would rather take group fitness classes, this is also a great option for comprehensive training that usually even includes flexibility training. On page 129, there's a special strength program for the feet that you can do often, and it doesn't require any special equipment.

Foot strength training is especially important if you have become accustomed to landing on the heel instead of using the foot's natural spring. If you have the time and motivation, you should also do the jump training. Jump training makes you stronger while improving muscle elasticity, and it allows you to run with lower energy consumption (see more on page 134). Just keep in mind that the load when you land is double that of when you run. Therefore it's important to only jump on soft ground and to learn a good landing technique.

Another good way to train the leg's ability to push is running up hills. Select a slope no steeper than you're able to run with a reasonably relaxed running stride. This makes the muscles work technically correctly while becoming stronger.

The muscles in the upper body are also important for your running. Above all, you need strong abdominals and back muscles that stabilize the torso so you can run with an upright posture and keep yourself from collapsing at the landing. Strong lower abdominals are also a requirement to be able to push forward with the hips in the run.

The role of the arms and shoulders in the running stride is to compensate for the movement of the leg on the opposite side of the body. When the right leg swings forward, the left arm and shoulder must do the same. Otherwise, the upper body rotates sideways, which costs a lot of unnecessary energy. Your arms should swing forward and backward with the elbow angled at roughly 90 degrees, with the possible exception of when the elbow turns in the rear position. Then the arm can be lowered slightly.

Runners rarely need to engage in any particular strength training for arms or chest muscles. A bad arm swing is almost always due to rigid and short muscles, not because they are too weak. In this context, it's time to warn you about exercises like push-ups and bench presses. Such training strengthens the muscles in the chest and arms; but this is something you don't have any use

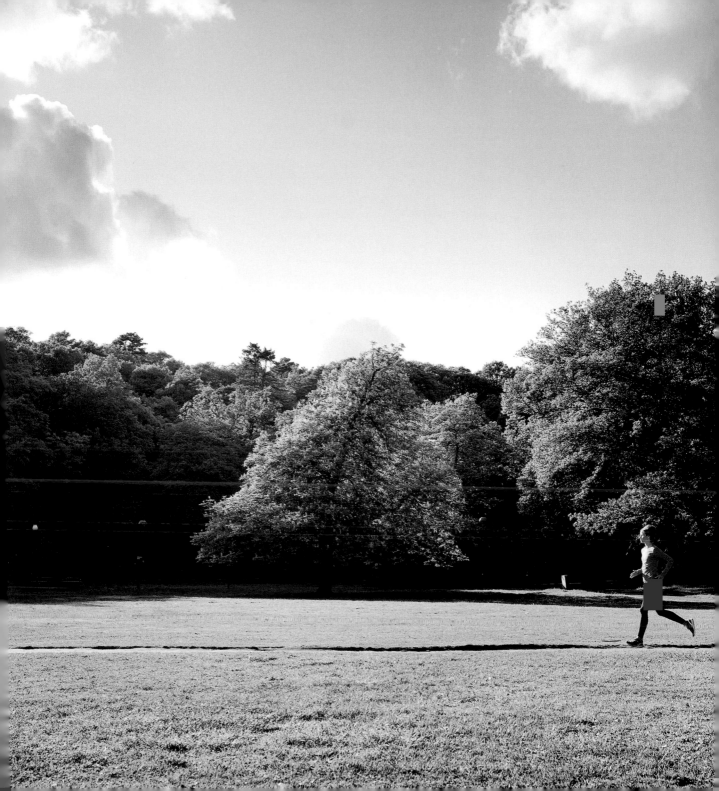

for when running because they don't create momentum or stabilize the torso. Instead, these exercises create the risk of shortened chest and shoulder muscles, which would impair the arm swing and posture.

Flexibility: a must for muscle strength

Your muscles' ability to develop force does not only depend on how strong they are. If you want to get the full effect of a muscle's work when running, that muscle must also have a certain length or elasticity to it. Too short hip flexors, hamstrings, or buttock muscles limit the legs' strides and make the running stride energy inefficient.

This doesn't mean that you have to run like Usain Bolt to get to an efficient running style. Sprint runners lift their knees at a 90-degree angle toward the hip and swing their arms almost halfway around the shoulder joint. That running technique costs too much energy for long distances and becomes wasteful and inefficient after only a few minutes. Think instead of Haile Gebrselassie—his movements are not as grand as Bolt's, but compared to an average distance runner the motions of his legs and arms are bigger, more powerful, and more relaxed. In return he gets a longer stride without expending more energy.

Your muscles need to be both strong and flexible to function optimally. But flexibility isn't just important for getting more power in your muscles. There's also an obvious correlation between how flexible your muscles are and how relaxedly you run. The latter is very important in endurance sports where you must reduce the build-up of lactic acid in the muscles by moving more relaxedly.

The disadvantage of rigid and short muscles is that they prevent you from having an efficient running style and they build up lactic acid faster. Limited flexibility also creates imbalances in the body that increase the risk of overloading a muscle.

You can improve flexibility primarily by stretching and muscle elongation. The difference between

> **❝ There's also a clear correlation between how flexible your muscles are and how relaxedly you run. ❞**

the methods is that stretching is static, while in elongation exercises you move back and forth toward the muscle's extended position. The benefit of elongation is that it increases blood circulation at the same time as it lengthens the muscles. Elongation is therefore better suited for warm-up. Almost all stretches can be performed as elongation, such as walking on the heels and forward or sideways swinging of the legs.

If elongation is most appropriate prior to the run, then stretching is preferable afterward. Stretching has a larger elongating effect, but it does require the muscles to be warm. With the help of stretching, tired and shortened muscles can regain their former length. Many also feel that stretching immediately after a tough workout reduces muscle soreness and makes you recover faster.

Change the rhythm and get stronger

Have you heard of eccentric movement? Or muscle elasticity?

Both concepts are about how to extract more energy from the muscles by training and running smarter. For a long distance runner there's a lot to gain here. And they're actually major factors in the Kenyan running wonder.

First, a little more about how your muscles work. When you run, the muscles shift between two phases in each running stride—engaged and relaxed. When the muscle is inactive it gets pulled apart and when it works it contracts to produce power. The muscle acts like a rubber band: it requires an external force to pull it apart, while it shrinks by its own power. An example is when the Achilles tendon and the calf muscles are pulled apart as a result of the bended ankle in the landing, after which they shrink and create power during the push-off phase.

When muscles are pulled apart—like in the calf muscles—they are not passive, but react by trying to curb the force that stretches them. The deceleration process is called eccentric and is very important in running. Research shows that muscles develop considerably more power when they are working to curb external forces, compared to when they contract under their own power. The difference is huge—up to 40 percent.

A concrete example to show how it works: imagine you are standing with stretched legs and a heavy

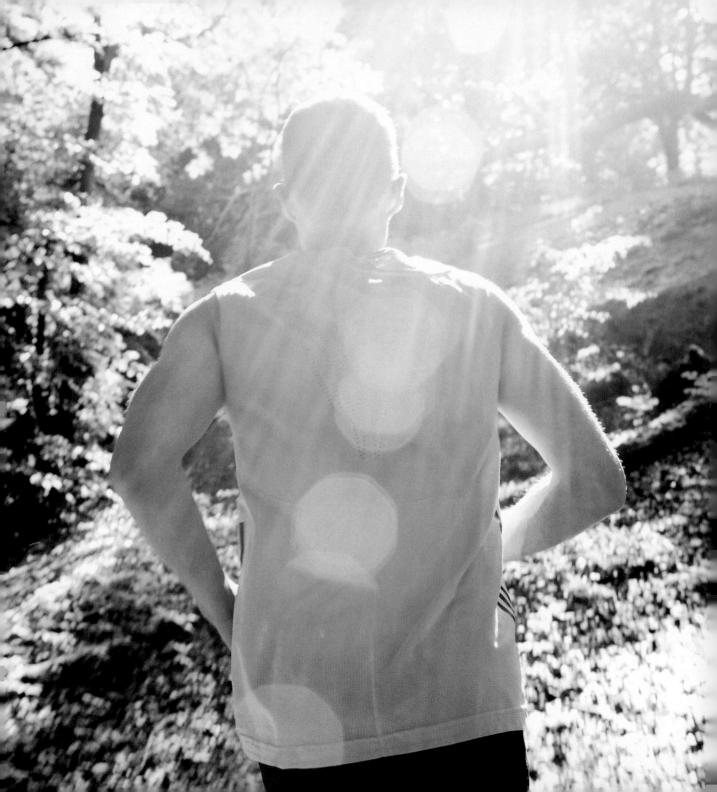

barbell on your shoulders. Despite the load, you will probably manage to bend your legs a bit without dropping the bar. However, it becomes much harder to move from the bent position to stretch your legs out again. This is because the tensors at the front of the thigh are much stronger when they work to decelerate on the way down than when they contract to develop power on the way up.

If you change the rhythm when you do strength training, you can easily make these muscles stronger by decelerating the phase. Instead of doing sit-ups, squats, and other dynamic exercises the usual way, working on the way up and resting on the way down, you change between the sets—go up quickly and then go slowly downward every other time. This way you train the muscles in an eccentric way and become up to 40 percent stronger.

If you count to four you will get a good rhythm. On "one" you work quickly up and then you are so slow on the way back down you have time to count "two-three-four" before the rebound. You'll notice right away if you've done it right because the exercise becomes considerably more strenuous when you load on the way down.

One advantage of being stronger in the decelerating phase is that your muscles become more elastic—they become better at slowing external forces that want to pull them apart. In the next paragraph, you can read why this ability is so important for your running endurance. Before that, we can conclude that the muscles' decelerating training also prevents injuries. It's only in this phase that the tendon of the muscle is active and receives blood circulation, which is healing as overload often hurts the tendon. Physiotherapists take advantage of this effect when they treat muscle ruptures and other overuse injuries. One example is the troublesome Achilles tendon, which is cured by so called negative toe raises where you work on the damaged tendon on the way down and on the way up you use the other leg's healthy Achilles tendon.

Muscle elasticity—the key to lower oxygen consumption

Muscle elasticity is one of the most energy-smart things the body has to offer. With it you can reduce oxygen consumption by 25 percent when running longer distances, which of course has a crucial impact on speed.

If you think the concept of elasticity and deceleration forces seems complicated, then you should know that it's something that comes automatically with good running technique. The Kenyan runners' sovereign ability to use their muscles' elasticity is one of the main reasons for their success, and they have gained it by running thousands of miles barefoot, thereby breeding a natural running style.

This is how elasticity works: When a muscle is working in a decelerated way it gets charged with energy that doesn't cost anything because it's kinetic energy that is formed by an external force pulling the muscle apart. The great thing about elastic energy is that it's free and can be stored and used a moment later when the muscle contracts to develop power. This is exactly what happens when the foot lands on the ground—the Achilles tendon is stretched a little and charged with energy, which it uses in the push-off phase. No less than 35 percent of the energy that the tendon consumes is reusable, "free" kinetic energy.

To create elastic energy in the muscles you need to run with a broad enough range of motion that pulls apart the muscles just before they produce power. It requires some flexibility and a well-coordinated running stride where the muscles alternate between activity and relaxation.

You improve muscle elasticity by technical training where you learn to lengthen the running stride just enough by doing jump and strength training exercises. When you skip, the load is increased in comparison to running on the ground, and this is because the force that pulls apart the muscles in the landing is stronger.

Technique

Powerful and elastic muscles are a requirement for good running economy. To reach an efficient and energy-saving running technique, your muscles also must be well coordinated.

This is where the brain enters the picture.

The ability to run with low energy consumption is all about doing it correctly and moving properly. It's not something you can influence with fitness training. Such training focuses on the heart and the body's transport of oxygen, but efficient running is dependent on the cooperation between the muscles and the brain. The difference between practicing cardio and practicing technique is the same as the difference between focusing on intensive effort rather than focusing on correct movements. Therefore, completely different rules apply to technical training than to cardio training. The way to more efficient running technique is through relaxation and good cooperation between the brain and muscles, and those are the two qualities that are prevented if you focus too much on "no pain = no gain."

When it comes to increasing your oxygen uptake, you have to push it to make gains. The bigger the load you put on the circulatory system (within reasonable limits), the greater the effect. But if you want to learn how to run more energy efficiently, then it's no doubt that "too much pain = no gain". One can also express this by saying that you will become a better runner if you learn to force it less when you run.

Yes, you read that right. Force it a little less, or "do less = achieve more". Anyone who has ever done any coordination-demanding activities such as golf, tennis, or dancing knows that it's not productive to push it fully all the time. Technical training is about reprogramming the brain, and in order to do so, the brain must be receptive and the physical load can't be too heavy.

> ❝ **The difference between practicing technique and cardio is also the difference between doing things correctly and forcing them.** ❞

Start with the basics

In order to learn how to run with smarter running technique, you need to adjust your speed to where you are at technically. It's only when you can perform a motion in a relaxed manner that it will come automatically, and then you can work up to performing it at full speed.

If you start with standing and walking exercises, then it's easier to find the correct body position. Next, try to master the position when you are in motion. Take it a little slower than usual and train yourself to find what feels right during your regular runs. That way, you train cardio and your technique simultaneously. Obviously, the cardio effect will be slightly less the first few times, but once you learn to do it correctly, your speed will increase without you having to force it more. You get more power from the same amount of energy. You can, of course, do tough cardio workouts in parallel and, gradually, with even better running technique.

The increase in speed you get with a more efficient running style lasts longer than what you can achieve with a few weeks or months of intensive interval training. Another advantage of technical training is that you don't need to force yourself until you taste blood. Rather, the challenge is to concentrate on doing it correctly, which requires that you be highly motivated and reasonably well-rested when you exercise. For learning, it's optimal to train your technique frequently, preferably two or three times per week, in order for the cooperation between the brain and muscles to establish itself quickly.

By improving your technique you gain a better awareness of your body, allowing you to concentrate on technique rather than exerting yourself more when you become fatigued. If you think about relaxing your shoulders to reduce the tension that restricts arm swing, then you can keep a higher pace for a longer time. And each time you do it, it becomes easier to find that relaxed mode.

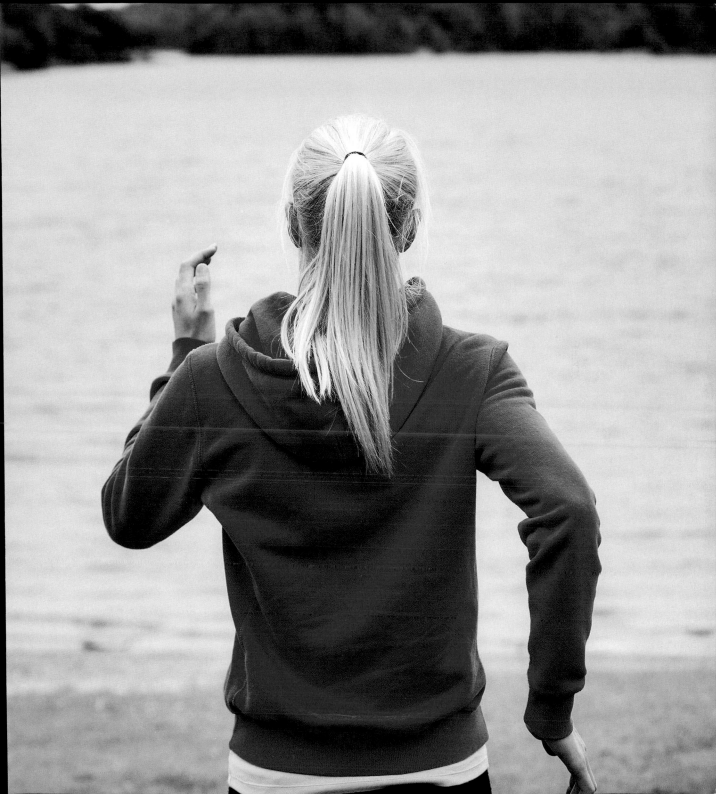

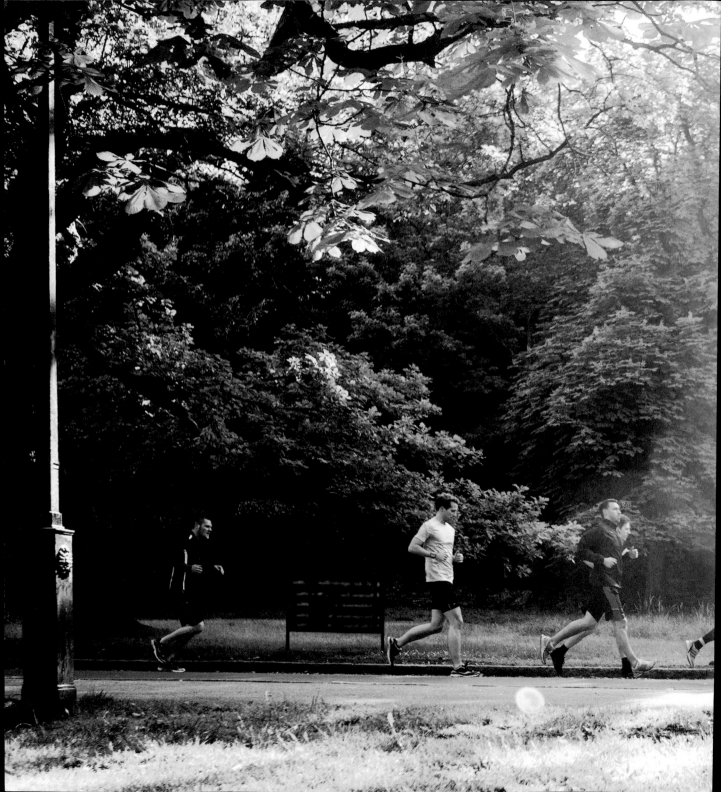

CHAPTER 3.

THE WAY TO FASTER RUNNING

3.

SPORTS ARE ALL ABOUT MOVING AS EFFICIENTLY AS POSSIBLE. Whether you play soccer, throw the javelin, or run a half marathon, you must customize your movement pattern for that particular sport to get the maximum out of your capacity.

The ideal standard for running is to run as fast as possible and consume as little energy as possible (that means a good running economy). You can't improve that quality with cardio training. Your physical fitness only determines how much energy you can turn over, not how good you are at using that energy.

The ability to run efficiently is something you can learn just like most other abilities. No one buys expensive golf equipment and plays regularly without worrying about whether or not he or she hits the ball. It only becomes fun when you learn how to hit the ball where you want it to go. It's just the same way when

you run—with more appropriate technique, your running will give you more.

It's no coincidence that the word "technique," which comes from the Greek, has its roots in terms like skill and proficiency. Running technique determines how good a runner you are. Regardless of fitness level, a more efficient running stride makes you keep your body in the right position so you can run at a higher speed even after fatigue sets in.

Good endurance requires an efficient running style. It's that simple. And running technique is something you can always improve, in contrast to fitness, which can only be improved up to a certain point. Best off are the runners who start working seriously on their technique at an early age. Just look at the Kenyans, who run with strong feet and efficient technique thanks to years of barefoot running during their youth.

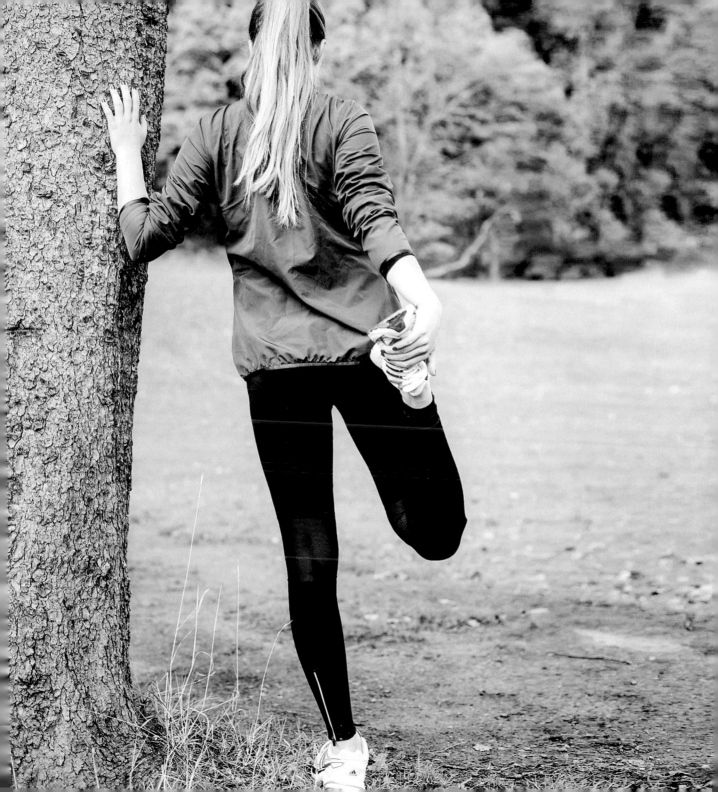

Your running stride starts in the brain

When you're training your technique, you need to use your brain more. Partly because you're exercising the brain's ability to control the muscles, and partly because you can make the learning easier through mental exercise. This is much easier than it sounds as you will realize later in this book.

One thing you'll need to learn is that you should think about how you run. During a regular run you can focus on your technique a few times per kilometer. Pretty soon you'll notice that the run is not very difficult and has become considerably less tiring, simply because you're focusing on moving correctly. Yes, it's actually more fun to run when you're concentrating on controlling your running technique. You get about the same satisfaction from running as many people say they get from cross-country skiing. When the thoughts are focused on getting the technique right, feelings of presence and relaxation increase, and you stop thinking about how long you still have left to run or how tired you feel.

The brain controls your running style, and it tells the muscles what to do via the nervous system.

Because there is a great variation in energy consumption, strides can look different. Therefore it's coordination—the cooperation between the brain and the muscles—that you have to improve if you want to reduce your energy consumption. Good coordination means that the "right" muscles are working at every step of the running stride while the opposing muscles are relaxed. This way you remove all the brakes and instead maximize the muscles' elastic energy. It also means your muscles are working with more balance, which reduces the risk of injury.

The interaction between the brain and the muscles works this way: when a movement should be performed, nerve cells in the cerebral cortex send signals to the appropriate muscles. Each nerve cell activates a large number of muscle cells, and a nerve cell with the associated muscle cell is called a motor unit. The goal of training your technique is to program the new motor units that make your running more economical.

Technical practice is powered by entirely different principles than cardio and strength training. The main difference is that the focus is to run as technically correctly as possible, not to maintain a certain speed. This is why the technique program is based on slow movements in order to gradually move toward faster running.

Take it easy

For some runners, it can feel like a workout hasn't done anything unless you get really tired. But when you're learning how to run more efficiently, you are training your brain and it becomes about creating new communication channels in the nervous system—in contrast to cardio running, which trains the heart, lungs, and blood vessels. If the learning intake is to work, then you must perform the movement correctly, which is facilitated by a more sedate pace, just like when you throw a dart, practice a dance step, or do something else where your coordination is challenged.

If it feels tricky to hold back on the pace, then you can think about the goal—by running slower and with more control, you will later have a completely different distribution of your fitness. You'll bring a new dimension to your ability, which will improve your running capacity in the long-term much more than if you're always pushing hard.

Subsequently, when you run more efficiently, you'll discover that

> **❝ With a better running economy, you will run 1,000-meter intervals about 10–20 seconds faster without having to push yourself harder than you did before. ❞**

easier running does not mean you're going slower. With a better running economy, you will run 1,000-meter intervals about 10–20 seconds faster without having to push yourself harder than you did before. Another pleasant discovery is that you can maintain a higher pace during the 10 kilometer run. You'll notice that you run faster because you don't struggle with tension against your own body. Instead, your body is with you, and you feel much better when running. Doesn't that sound great? It is.

Programming a running stride

When you move, you're normally not aware of what's happening in the body. If you lift a chair or walk up a flight of stairs, you don't really think about which muscles are working. The movement is automatic because the brain has been taught—the movement has been automated in the part of the brain that's outside of your consciousness. The neural pathways that go from the brain to the muscles are connected via neurons in the spinal cord, and you don't need to make any conscious choices.

Technical running's biggest challenge is transforming your training into an automatic motion. You've become used to running a certain way—maybe with your torso tilted forward. To relearn the movement and push your hips forward, you'll need to think actively about what you're doing, otherwise you'll automatically run the way you're used to. It's only when you're performing the new movement that your brain builds new connections between the nerve and muscle cells.

Learning a new movement works in much the same way that you program a computer. The brain installs new routines to replace the old. The difficulty of running in a new way is caused by the fact that the old links between the brain and muscles are stronger than the new ones. Your body "wants" to run as it's accustomed to run. Therefore, in order to install the new program—meaning the movement—you must perform the new movement with technical precision. Do it slowly and correctly, rather than halfway correctly with more repeats. Each time you repeat a movement incorrectly, it becomes even more difficult to reprogram it.

This is the same way it works in all kinds of coordinative challenges—whether you're learning to dance salsa, juggle a ball, or skateboard. Even if you concentrate, it's hard to do it right before the new neural pathways between the brain and muscles have been established. But practice helps you to improve. The brain becomes better at what it does practice and worse at what it does not. Therefore, it becomes easier to run correctly the more you practice it.

The length of time it takes to learn how to run efficiently at full speed depends on how often you practice your technique and how careful you are, especially when you implement the new movement into your running style. A common mistake is that you practice technique before you run, in the form of various exercises, and then forget to apply that technique to the actual running. But the reason to practice having high hips, low shoulders, or an active ankle is to be able to use the movement in the running stride. If you can't do it there, then there's no reason to practice your running technique at all.

Therefore, try as quickly as possible to apply the correct basic posture in your regular running, even if it slows you down at the beginning. With the help of a mental trigger (see page 63), you reinforce the learning intake. In the beginning you may still be tempted to push yourself the old way, but once you discover that it costs less energy, that you can actually go faster by focusing on your running technique, and that this makes it easier to run correctly, you will become a much better runner.

Develop your own running technique

The goal of this book is to teach runners of all levels to run more economically. With the help of the unique training program in chapters 6–8, which was developed in cooperation with leading experts on learning and running, you can create your own workouts.

All learning is facilitated by moving from easy to difficult. Therefore, the method is based first on the fact that you learn some still standing

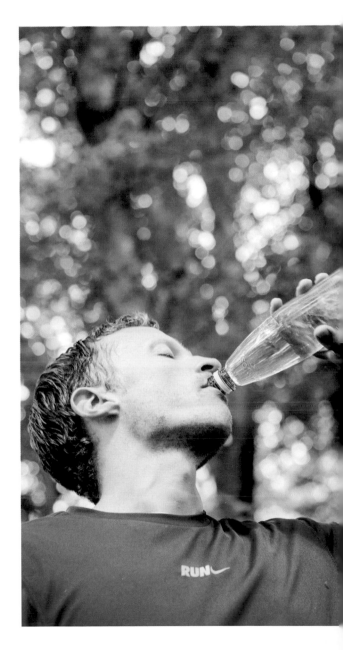

Your brain wants training

Practicing your technique is about programming your brain. It's also a type of exercise that has become increasingly important in sports. This is largely because of the enormous advances in brain research made in the past ten years. The knowledge evolves so quickly that there's talk of a revolution in the perception of the human brain.

The key concept is plasticity; the brain is malleable. Unlike previously thought, the brain can both form new cells and reorganize itself with new networks throughout your lifetime. You're not born with a certain amount brain cells that then decrease as you get older.

The consequence of this new research is that everything that is controlled by the brain is considered much more changeable than was previously understood—movements, behaviors, yes even the human aging process. Research shows that older people who regularly solve crossword puzzles, study new languages, play music, or spend time on other cognitive challenges almost completely stop the deterioration of their brain's faculties. The reason for this is that the brain will continue to form new connections between neurons as long as it receives stimulation, no matter if you are fifteen or eighty-five years old.

The advances within brain research pave the way for new training methods. It would be very strange if they didn't. Why should we train like we did thirty or fifty years ago when today's knowledge points to completely different results?

For example, today there is computer technology that offers a detailed analysis of running stride. Within a few years, it will be an important tool for runners who have the knowledge to interpret their movements and correct them. This book gives you those skills.

Awareness of the importance of technique has also reached team sports, such as soccer. In such a complex sport, players must have endurance, strength, and technique. But in terms of talent, the focus is currently on technique and on the training of the brain. A survey of the top European clubs show that all of them prioritize qualities that have to do with the brain, such as ball technique and game knowledge, because those characteristics set the limit for how good a soccer player can become, not physical factors such as physical fitness and strength.

positions and slow movements, which you gradually implement in a faster running style. Thanks to the fact that the initial exercises are easy to evaluate by using either a mirror or a film camera, you know when you're doing it right and how it should feel. That is the feeling you then bring with you in to your run.

If you want to study your running technique, you can run on a treadmill in a room with mirrors or let someone film you from the side so you can see the way your foot lands, your posture, and hip position.

The best proof that you are running more efficiently you obviously get in the form of improved time. Even if it takes a while before you're able to use the technique at full speed, you can still get measurable feedback at an early stage on how your technique is developing by taking the tests in Chapter 10. For instance, select one or more of the tests and do them once every month. Then you can follow how your stride length, foot landing, and running economy develop over time.

Focus on one thing at a time

A basic rule when training your technique is to focus on one thing at the time. This is because practicing your technique is a brain exercise, and because your short-term memory has a limited capacity, you can't really concentrate on two things at once. Just think about how difficult it is to type a text message at the same time as you're driving a car. And how dangerous driving becomes when something else suddenly requires your attention.

If you try to think of several technical details at the same time, they will compete for your attention. Then it will be much harder to perform the movement correctly, and there is a great risk that you will consolidate erroneous movements. This is why dance classes always start by practicing only the leg movements. Only when the legs have learned the dance steps can you concentrate on the arms and torso. The order in running is different, as you will discover later. However, it's just as important to concentrate on one section at the time. You can't think about hip position at the same time as paying attention to your foot landing.

In order to be able to focus on one element of running at a time, we have divided the technical training into three parts—hip work, posture, and foot landing. The idea is that you should stick to one of the subsections for a few weeks or months—depending on how long it takes before the technical training starts to deliver. Remember that a more effective running stride requires changes in the communication between the brain and muscles, and it is no quick fix. But the effects are long-term.

Look at your own needs when choosing between the hips, shoulders, and foot landing. If you're unsure of what to prioritize, ask a friend to film your running style. If you're not accustomed to practicing running technique or are unsure of how to run, then it is best to start from the hip for an efficient running style. If you have poor posture and/or stiff shoulders, then it may be better to begin by focusing on the shoulders. If you're already running with an upright posture and pushing with the hips, then you can go straight to working on the foot landing. But keep in mind that you must have strong ankles to be able to land and work properly with your feet.

Even if you only train one part of your technique, you will see the effects on the whole body.

This is because the running stride is a whole, an interaction of many muscles, where a correction in one part affects the rest of the body.

With more upright posture and relaxed shoulders, the hips will fall into a better position. And when you run with your hips more tilted upwards-forward, you will automatically land with your feet under the body rather than in front of it, which makes the landing faster—even if you're still landing on the heel.

Find your trigger!

Technical training and mental training have a lot in common. In both cases, it's about taking cues from the brain to make the body perform better. Among elite athletes, it's common to use a trigger from mental exercise—a thought that creates the right feeling in your body. It's a simple trick that you can also use to run more efficiently, especially when you are transferring what you learned from technique exercises into your run. But remember that your trigger should be an image and not a word or a sentence.

When learning new movements, a picture is worth a thousand words. In contrast to words, we receive images with the brain's creative right side and it facilitates learning. Just think about how children learn—by watching others do something and then imitating them. In adulthood, we work the same way, even though we've become used to describing and understanding through words and analysis instead of images.

When the brain works from an image it does not need extra effort to analyze what is happening, which allows the body to learn a new movement much faster. In one experiment, some students from Sweden's School of Sport and Health Sciences went slalom skiing while thinking about different things. They performed the worst when they thought about five different things in their technique. They performed the best when they focused on a single image of a perfect performance.

You may pick your picture from any exercise in technical programs. The important thing is that it is a clear picture of the ideal movement or pose that illustrates your goal. When you focus on the image you've chosen, you send out information to every cell in the body, and in that way you affect the way you run. If you practice your hip technique, then it can be an image of the hips being located at the front and pulling the rest of the body forward. If you're focusing on the upper body, then you might think of an image of low and relaxed shoulders. Or, if you're practicing the foot landing, then you may imagine yourself landing on the front part of the foot. The most important thing is that the image is clear so you can think of it when you run.

Once you get used to running in a new way, the communication between the brain and muscles increases. Then your inner image of the movement becomes more detailed, and you get more than one trigger for the same movement. For example, instead of having low shoulders as a trigger, it can also be that you have an internal image of upright posture and arms that gently accompany the running stride without shortening the leg stride. This is something that is very useful, because it's easier to run technically correctly when you vary between different images of the same goal.

Variation is important for all learning, like when children learn to write, when you practice a new language, or practicing to run with better technique. Increased variation gives the brain more stimulation and it can form more links to the right motor units. Consequently, more paths are created that lead to the goal—a more efficient running stride.

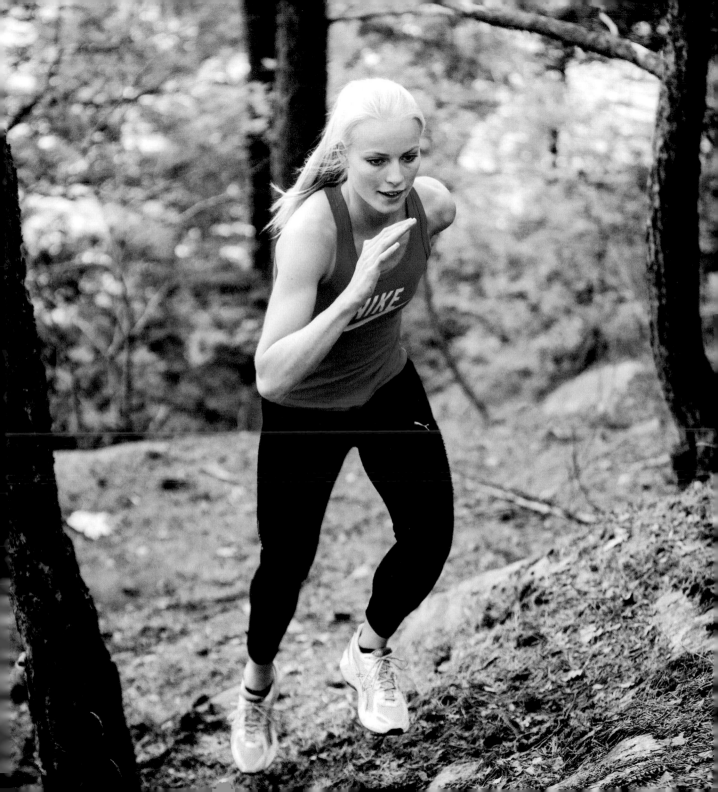

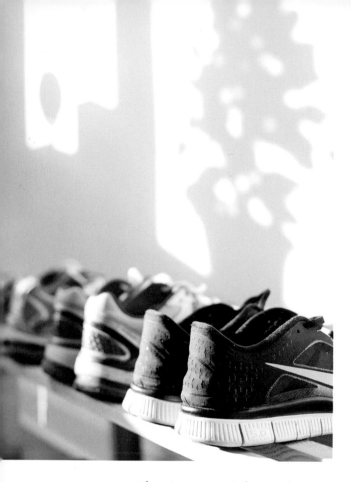

ways. The more of the exercises you're able to perform properly, the faster and better you learn to run with the right hip position at full speed. But remember, it is better to master one exercise than to perform five halfway and sloppy.

Variation doesn't just stimulate the brain to form new connections—the training will be more fun for you, as well, which helps you to learn new things.

Use your trigger in competitions

If you participate in a race or competition, you can obviously benefit from being able to control your technique. In practice, this means you can access a higher gear. In the critical stages, as in hills or when you start to feel fatigued, you can counteract the slowing down by focusing on your technique. Instead of giving into fatigue and stumbling onward, which only increases energy consumption, use your trigger and focus on, for example, keeping an upright posture. In the same way, you can, of course, use the trigger to raise the pace if you want to keep up with someone who speeds up or when sprinting to the finish line.

There's no contradiction between variation and focusing on one thing at the time. When practicing a certain technical element, it's only to your advantage to do it in several different ways. This is why the program contains many different exercises that train the same thing. Switch up the exercises as often as you can. For example, you can practice the hip position by standing, walking, jumping, and running in different

What happens is that your running technique immediately gets trimmed and you get faster without increasing your energy consumption. It's an incredible feeling to able to increase speed without forcing yourself.

But you also gain mental benefits from focusing on your running technique. Anyone who has competed knows how easy it is to get stressed out by the crowds and all the other competitors in the competition. In the worst case scenario, this impairs your performance. The chances are that you're tempted to run too fast at the start of the run, and your muscles fill with lactic acid. Another danger is that in the seriousness of the moment, you run more tensely, with an inferior running economy. By running with

> **" It's an incredible feeling to able to increase speed without forcing yourself. "**

technique in focus, you can shut off all disturbing impressions in a race, just as in mental training where you turn to yourself and focus on how you ought to run. Then you won't easily become distracted by everything that happens around you. You'll know what is important in your running and know how to manage your body so you can enjoy it.

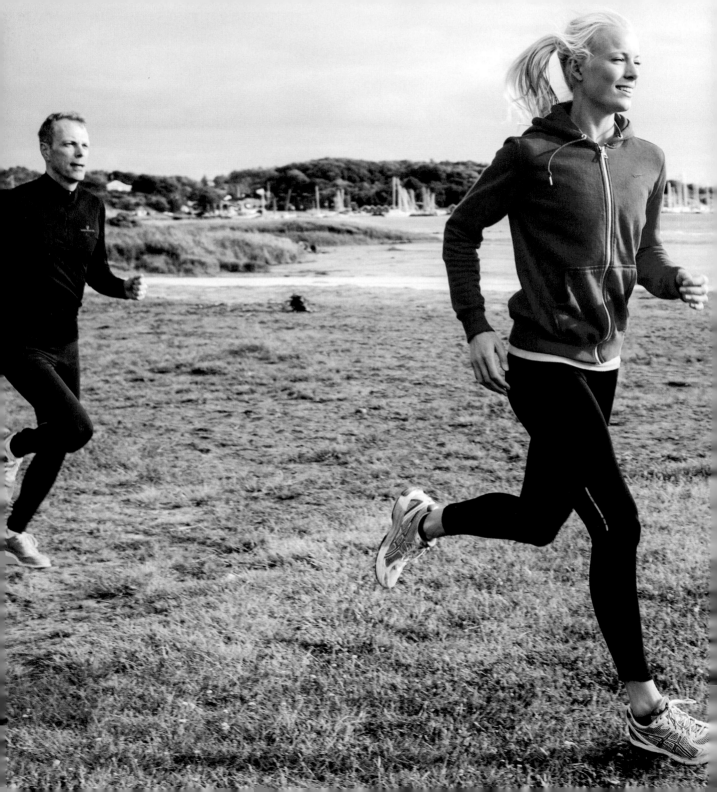

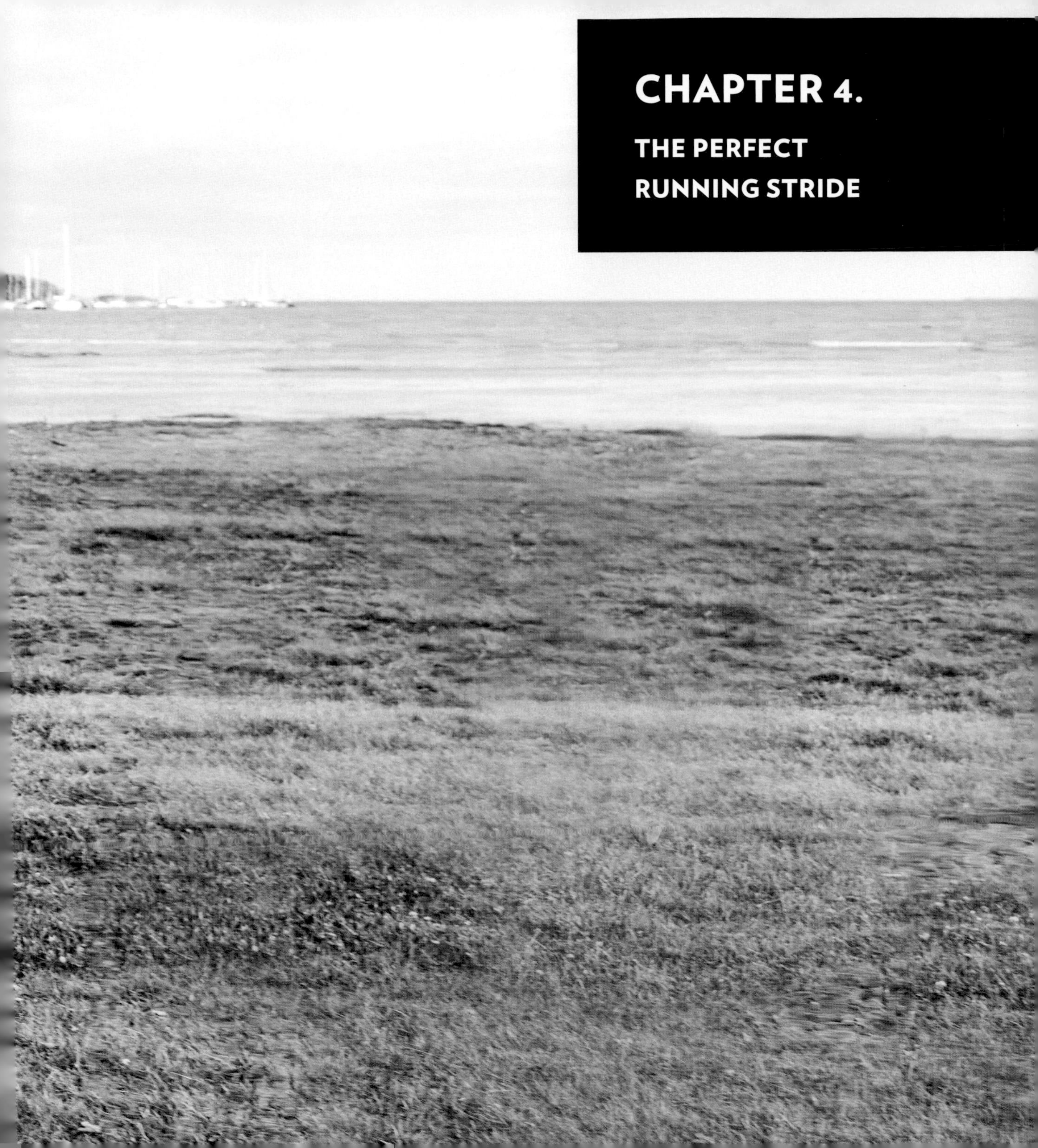

CHAPTER 4.

THE PERFECT RUNNING STRIDE

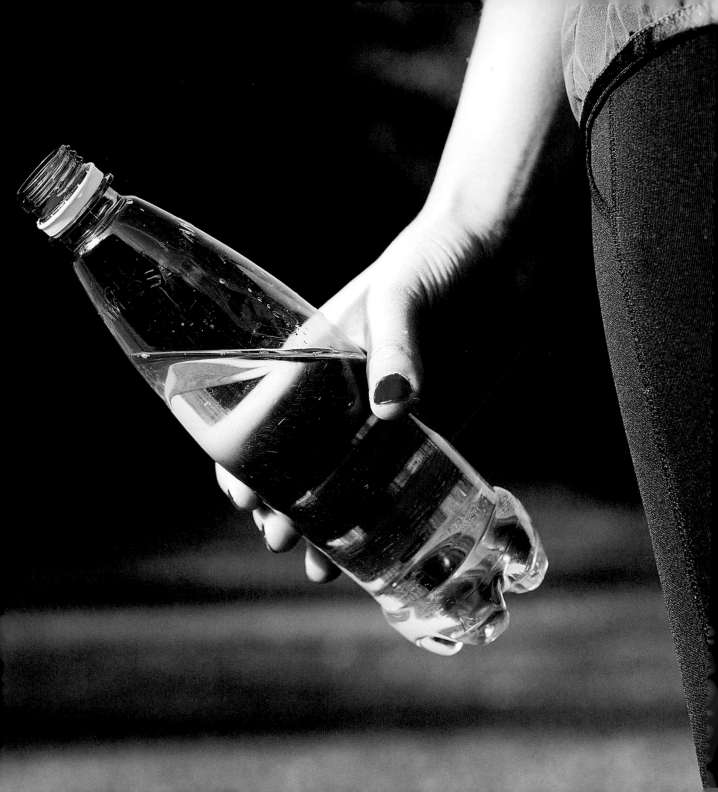

4.

EVERYONE HAS HIS/HER OWN PERSONAL RUNNING STYLE. You can study runners in any race and you will see how differently they all run. The variation is so vast because of differences in body composition, height and weight, and because running style is a combination of several movements in different joints—how much the upper body leans forward, if the hips are stretched or arched, how long the arm swing is, where on the foot you land, and so on.

But differences in running styles don't just look different when we run. There is also a big difference in energy consumption, depending on how we run—this is why there can be a 30 percent difference in running economy between two runners who are in equally good shape. With effective running technique, one person can run 10 kilometers in 35 minutes, while his friend with the same oxygen uptake ability but with an energy-wasting running style takes 50 minutes to run the same stretch. This is equivalent to the difference in fitness between an elite runner and a decent exerciser.

The way to a better running economy is via changes in your running style—toward more efficient running technique. And to improve your running technique on your own, you need to have a good understanding of what a good running style looks like. In this chapter, you'll get the foundation that is required to use the exercise programs later in this book.

Improve technique, lower energy consumption

A good running technique has nothing to do with whether it looks attractive or ugly. The key is to keep energy consumption as low as possible and, to achieve that, you should run so that you take advantage of both gravity and the muscles' stored energy. As a bonus, you reduce your risk of injury by 50 percent. It's all about running relaxedly and naturally, about getting back to how you ran as a child. And you will get there by taking it easier and thinking more about how you are moving.

Running stride is based on certain basic movements. No one reaches the level of the world's elite without a good technique. You can be sure that all participants in an Olympic final of the 10,000-meter run push their strides forward from the hips, taking advantage of the elasticity of the muscles, and that they use their foot's natural spring every time they land on the ground.

The running styles at the highest levels also differ in details that do not compromise the foundation of running technique. Some runners may have a loftier arm swing than others or may run more tilted. As long as the arm swing is not stiff or short so that it restricts the leg's movements, it may have a variety of appearances. And it's fine to tilt the upper body more forward or backward as long as the hips are forward in the run.

A runner in the 1990s got a lot of attention for his seemingly excessively backward-tilted upper body-running style; this was Michael Johnson, world record holder in the 400 meters. Some looked at Johnson's running as a proof that running technique does not impact how fast you run. But, in-depth analysis of Michael Johnson's running style actually shows that he ran more upright than his competitors, but he did not break the essential technical requirements. Johnson ran with his hips at an upward-angled position, which made the power of the rapid foot landing push him forward. Moreover, the range of motion in his leg and arm swing was of equal size to that of the other high-level sprinters and this way he could use the muscle's elastic energy.

Three keys to the perfect running stride

The obvious differences in running styles—even among the most ambitious runners who run for exercise—are because many are careless about those simple and basic movements that are very important for running economy. We have several times discussed how common it is for people to land on the heel and roll over the foot, rather than using the foot's natural spring. Another common mistake is that one tilts the upper body forward instead of pushing the hips forward. The result is a "sitting" running style where the feet slow down the run, and a lot of energy is wasted. In the training programs later in this book, we have borrowed heavily from sprinting and adapted it for long distance runners. It's about technical details that make your stride faster without expending more energy, like running with a more rapid foot landing, pushing with the hips and relaxing your shoulders so that the arm swing becomes synchronized with the movements of the legs.

Sprinting has gone significantly further than middle and long distance running in terms of practicing running technique. It's because physical fitness has no significance when competing at short distances. It's all about muscles and technique, and therefore tremendous resources have been put into developing methods to run more efficiently. And even though there are differences—sprinting is about developing a lot of power in a short period of time, while middle and long distances are about running with a low energy consumption for a long period of time—the running stride based on the same principles of the body's levers and muscles works the same whether you run 100 meters or a marathon. This means that for long distance runners who want to run smarter and with lower energy consumption there is a lot to learn from sprinting.

The perfect running stride can be described as a movement where, by pushing the hips forward, the whole body weight moves forward and the feet land under the body and push it forward. An upright upper body facilitates the hips' forward tilting position. The fitness programs later in the book are based on different elements of the running stride:

» The hips should be angled upward and forward (Chapter 6)

» The shoulders should be low and relaxed (Chapter 7)

» The feet should land underneath the body and work actively on the ground (Chapter 8)

If you want to learn how to run more efficiently, you must use your personal running style as your starting point. You are probably doing some things correctly but need to improve on others. Therefore, you will get the most out of selecting one of the keys to the perfect running stride and focusing on it. Do you remember the message from Chapter 3? Learning works best if you concentrate on one thing at a time; but by developing one part of the stride—in the hips, shoulders, or feet—everything is affected.

Hips—push yourself forward

Running is all about providing power to the ground, which is the power you get when you push off from the ground, driving the body forward. To get as much benefit as possible from the power, tilt your hips up (away with the arch) and let them push the stride forward. The body's center of gravity is actually in the hips, and when you run with the hips in such a position, it takes up the maximum power from the push-off and creates more movement forward—you get a longer stride without it costing you more energy.

A comparison with moving a stalled car shows how important the push-off is for the run. It's much easier to move your car if you push it from behind rather than trying to pull the car behind you with a rope. In the same way, it's much easier to run if you push the hips forward and let the push-off power come from behind. If you instead run "sitting" with arched hips, you get no help from the push-off and are forced to land with your feet in front of you in order to pull yourself forward, which is a waste of energy equivalent to pulling a car behind you instead of pushing it forward.

The hips' up-facing position is the most important part of an efficient running style. It makes you

» use the push-off power optimally

» create a forward falling movement with each step

» use the energy from the muscle elasticity

» hit the ground with a faster foot landing

» run more relaxedly

When you push your hips forward, the body's center of gravity lands so far forward that in addition to the push-off power, on every step you also get a controlled falling reflex that increases the speed of the leg's forward swing. That way, you use the weight of your own body to speed ahead instead of using your legs to pull yourself forward, which makes the running stride much more efficient. The falling reflex also reduces the strain on your knees and spine by up to 50 percent compared to a running style where you land with your foot in front of the body and pull yourself forward.

The two advantages of tilted hips—the falling reflex and more power in the push-off—give you a longer running

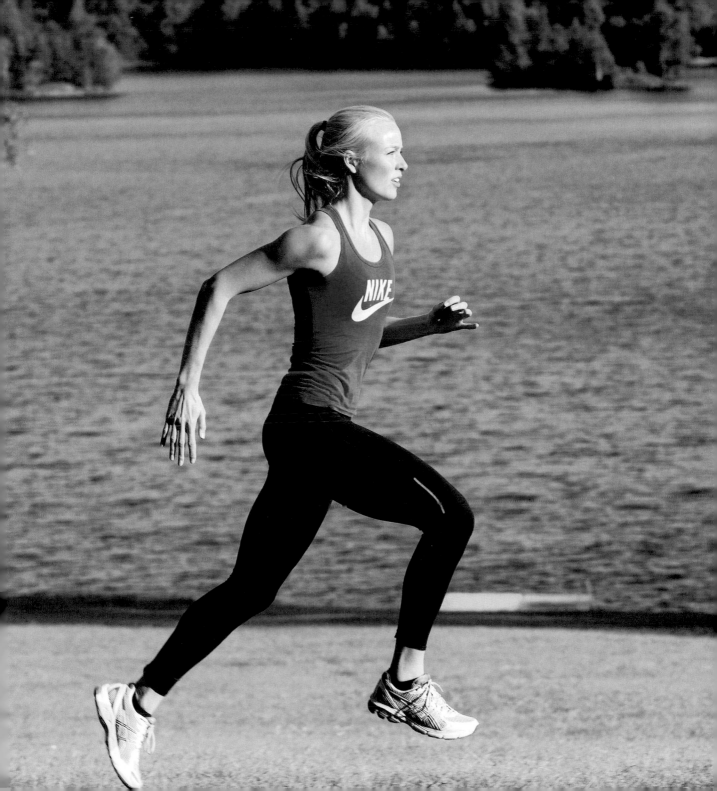

stride without costing more energy. If you extend the stride by 10 cm, which is a reasonable improvement, you run 18–20 meters more every minute. After a kilometer, the difference is up to 100 meters. This corresponds to a reduction of almost half a minute per kilometer or 5–10 minutes in a half marathon without having to train more cardio. Actually, the effect of a more forward hip position is even greater, because you can also better use the elasticity of the muscles.

If you actively work the hips, you also lay the foundation for other important elements of the run. It may be impossible to land with your feet under your body if your hips are not far enough ahead. Therefore, you'll automatically get a more rapid foot landing just by correcting the position of your hips.

Another benefit of running with active hips is that the muscles in your legs, buttocks, and trunk will be loaded more naturally as a result of the fact that the body is in the right position. It makes your running more relaxed while reducing the risk of injury.

Find the right position

The basic position in running is based on your tilted and upward-facing hips. Try to see how easy or difficult it is for you to get there: stand with your legs a shoulder width apart and with your upper body upright. Start with arching and then do the opposite, tense your buttocks and tilt the bottom of your hips, the pelvis, forward and upward. In this position, tilt yourself forward with your hips and torso in a straight line until your heels lift from the ground, leaving only the front part of your foot on the ground. This is the optimal position for running that you should always strive for. If you are doing it correctly, the hips should be so far forward that you are on the verge of triggering the falling-reflex.

To be able to run with the hips in this position requires some strength and mobility. You need to have strong abdominals that keep the pelvis in place while reducing the arch in the lower back. And you need to be sufficiently flexible in the hip flexors. Therefore, we've included strength and flexibility exercises in the training program for the hips.

Once you have learned to stand with your hips pushed forward, go ahead and practice the pose in motion—walk or run in place by lifting your knees and landing with the front part of your foot straight under the body. Then press your hips forward and feel how you fall forward, but continue to land with your feet under your body so that your hips push the motion forward. It is a big eye-opener the first time you feel the hips push the body forward. Once you have found that feeling, a lot of the work is done because the movement is natural and is easy to return to.

A good exercise to teach your hips their job is to tow a workout friend (see page 106). Try to feel the difference in power when you press forward with the hips compared with when you drag yourself forward with the feet and legs. You can also discover the difference when you walk.

Instead of landing with your foot in front of you and pulling yourself forward, try to land with your feet under your body while you angle your hips upward and push them forward as in the basic position mentioned previously. When you do it correctly, the speed increases without it costing you any extra energy.

You can also practice the power from the hip on hills. When the hill rises, you are slowed down by gravity and therefore you spontaneously land with the feet under your body in order to push yourself forward. Take that feeling and try to do the same on a flat surface. When going downhill, when gravity gives you extra speed, it's common to brake by pulling back the hips so your feet land in front of the body. Instead, try in a shallow downhill incline to land with your feet under your hips and feel how your whole body gets an extra boost. If you can transfer that feeling to your regular running, you have taken a big step toward a better running economy.

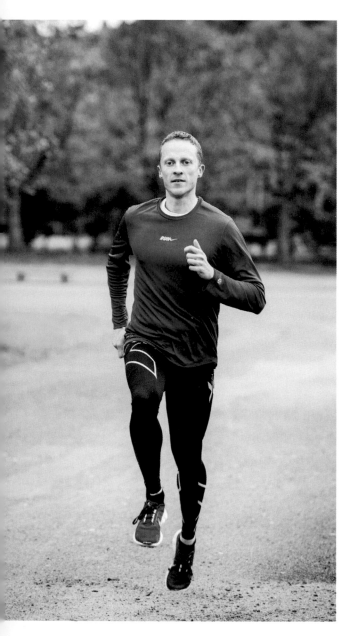

Extend your legs with the help of the hips

In addition to tilting your hips upward, you can also move the hip flexors in another way by lifting one hip upward and forward. The result is that the hip follows the leg through the stride forward and backward, and in this way extends the running stride.

You are probably already using this joint movement in your running stride, but if you train it, you can increase your hip's sideways motion and extend the stride further. The hip has the same effect on the running stride as the hub has on a bicycle wheel; it increases the length of your running stride for every extra centimeter you lift the hips sideways.

A good way to find the right feeling for the movement is to imitate a power walker. Feel how each hip follows the leg so that the step starts from the hips rather than the thighs. Try to lift the hip of the leg that is striding forward so the hip moves in a circular motion upward-forward-down-backwards.

Then when you run, you have to make the motion as large as possible while at the same time angling the hip in the basic position we described in the previous paragraph. It's not as difficult as it sounds—quite the opposite; with a forward tilted hip leading the movement forward, it's actually easier to raise and lower the hips sideways with the leg stride.

The hip's synchronized motion with the leg's stride is also important for your rhythm when running. When one hip turns in the front outer position, the other automatically slides forward in a constant flow. Runners who don't take advantage of this motion due to stiffness or poor coordination are not only missing out on a longer stride, but they also get a more spasmodic running style. In the training program system on page 104, there are strength and flexibility exercises that help you free the power of your hips and reduce the risk of locking your hips when fatigue comes.

Shoulders—don't let arm swing affect your stride

It's easy to think that the shoulders are not important in running, but tension in this part of the body is one of the most common obstacles to a good running style. Obviously, you run with the legs, but the shoulders' position affects both your arm swing and your posture, which has great significance for the running stride. Therefore, it may be good to examine what happens in the upper body when running.

To understand how important the shoulders and the posture are for your run, try to walk ten meters with a curved back and high, forward-tilting shoulders. Then compare that with what happens if on the way back you keep an elongated torso and low shoulders. With a more upright posture, the hips are pushed forward and that increases the length of the stride.

Relaxed shoulders:

» create good conditions for a proper arm swing

» help keep a good posture, which improves running economy

» can improve the oxygen uptake yield by increasing the lung capacity

The arms are attached to the shoulder sockets, and therefore it's your shoulders that determine how much of and how fast an arm swing you have. Unfortunately, it's very common—especially in people who played soccer or lifted weights from their early teenage years—to run with tense and high shoulders. Tense shoulders shorten the arm swing and automatically shorten the running stride, regardless of how you move your legs and hips. This is fine when you play soccer, as it's easier to get right up to the ball with a shorter step; but the problem is that as long as you don't do something about the shoulders, the stride remains equally short even when you run long distance. The disadvantage of a shortened step is that the push-off is not fully utilized, which means that you get a much more ineffective drive forward, and therefore the run becomes quite inefficient.

The ideal in running is a relaxed arm swing that is synchronized with the leg's movements. In practice, this means that the legs determine the speed and drive you forward in the run, while the arms gently accompany you by swinging at the same speed and with an equal range of motion.

If you want to find out whether your arms are restricting your running style, you can run with your hands on your neck (see the exercise on page 122). What happens is that when the legs do not need to consider the arm swing, the hips move more, and therefore the running stride is extended. The trick is to keep the momentum of the running stride when you bring your arms back down to swing again. Try to concentrate on making the arm swing adapt to the legs and running stride instead of limiting it.

For many runners it's an eye-opener to discover how the running stride is lengthened when your arms are not allowed to affect the leg's motion. Once you find that feeling, you can use it as a trigger to make the same movement in your regular running.

An upright posture makes you a better runner

Tense shoulders are usually caused by sitting still for too long. When you sit for a long period of time, the neck doesn't manage to hold up the head, and therefore you jerk forward and pull the shoulders upward and forward. The result is that the shoulders are in a position to reduce blood circulation and this makes them stiff and inflexible. Once this happens, you risk being stuck in a curved posture with high shoulders and a hunched back. You will then run with this same posture, and unfortunately, regular running will not help to correct it. Long distance running gives more endurance to the muscles, but for those who have

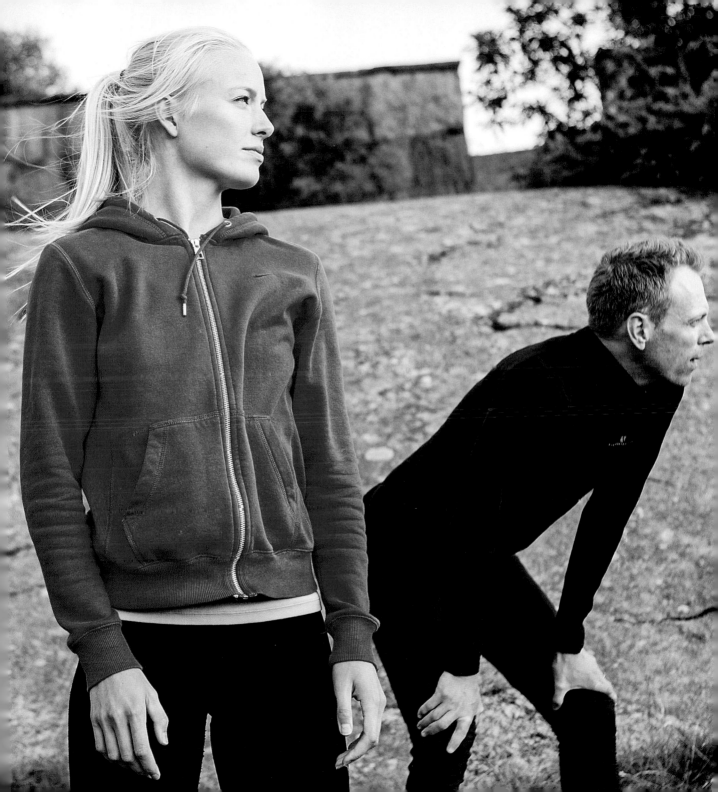

bad posture the running stride will remain uneconomical as long as nothing is done to fix the shoulders.

Your posture is very important for your running economy. If you run with an upright upper body to distribute weight evenly across the body and avoid overloading any joints or muscles, you will have a relaxed, natural, and energy-efficient run.

In order to have good posture, your shoulders must be low and relaxed, and then your upper body will stretch longer, and the hips will automatically tilt forward. A common error among runners is to do the opposite: lean the shoulders and chest forward so much that the hips fall backwards.

To push on forward when running is all about pushing the hips forward, not your chest.

It's optimal to run with the body in a vertical line, which means that it makes a straight line from the ear through the shoulders, hips, and knee down to the foot. It should feel like you have a string that holds up your head while stretching out the neck. For those who are stiff in the back and shoulders, it can be difficult to stand and almost impossible to run with this posture, but really, it is the most natural and functional posture—the one we have as children.

The feeling of an upright posture is important to have when you run.

The shoulders are a place where tension appears when fatigue sets in, which often leads to both a worsened posture and arm swing. However, if you learn to relax your shoulders, you can work to combat this.

To get a better posture and a more efficient arm swing, you must first become more flexible in the muscle that restricts the shoulder's movement and become stronger in the muscles that extend the upper back. This means you should exercise flexibility in the shoulders, chest muscles, and the neck muscles that lift and lower your shoulders. At the same time, strengthen the muscles around the shoulder blades (see program page 117). You don't need to be stronger in the chest and arm muscles, as strength training in those parts of the body will only reduce the flexibility in the shoulders.

The rewards of a better posture are not only a more efficient running style. Posture is a constant in your life, and this means that you will move more smoothly and with less effort in everything you do. Additionally, you'll look better and healthier with your shoulders shifted backwards and chest up.

Stretch yourself upright and get a better fitness

Good posture improves your running economy, but the fact is that it can also affect your physical fitness. This is because there's a relationship between posture and your breathing. Try taking deep breaths when you stand up with a straight back and low shoulders. Then, compare how it feels to breathe when you have a curved back and high forward-shifted shoulders. Bad posture closes the ribcage and makes the lungs work harder to breathe in air.

What happens when your shoulders are pulled back and your chest opens is that the lungs get more room to expand when they breathe in air. Since the lungs have less resistance when breathing, it's easier to breathe. This has a major effect in races because the lungs will devour up to 20 percent of the body's energy when forced to work harder than necessary. A better posture provides a better capacity for the respiratory muscles. How large the effect would be on your fitness depends on how good your posture is at the start, but there is no doubt that runners with poor posture have much to gain even fitness-wise when running in a more upright position.

> **" To push on forward when running is all about pushing the hips forward, not your chest. "**

Feet—use the natural springs

When running, it's important that each step has as short a contact with the ground as possible because each landing puts a brake on your speed. To meet the ground quickly, you must land on the front part of the foot. It doesn't matter that the heel touches the ground early in the contact, but in the push-off, the pressure should be on the arches of your feet. These are the muscles that allow the foot to act as a spring. The pressure of bodyweight loads the arches and the Achilles tendon with elastic energy when the foot meets the ground. In the momentum following the landing, the foot and calf develop a force that pushes you forward. If you instead land on the heel and roll forward on the foot, you completely miss out on the spring effect of the foot and the Achilles tendon, which makes the contact with the ground much longer. The foot landing is crucial to your running economy because running begins with the foot's contact with the ground.

With a good foot landing, you will

» run faster

» save energy

» increase the power of the push-off

» get better balance

» reduce the risk of injury in knees, hips, and back.

To be able to land on the front part of your foot, you have to land under the body. This requires that you run with your hips in a forward position. If your hips don't lead the movement forward, the foot will land in front of the body and you'll land on your heel. The problem with heel landing is not only that the contact with the ground takes more time, but also that you won't be able to take advantage of the natural spring in your feet and your running economy will be much worse.

If you are used to landing on your heels you have an awful lot to gain from learning to land on the front part of the foot instead. But two things are required to make the transition. First, you need to build strength in the feet and calves to cope with the increased load on the ankles, and then you must learn to run with your hips in a prominent position so that you land with your feet under the body.

Unburden the knees and back

In *Born to Run*, Christopher McDougall lays blame on the heel inserts of modern running shoes. When the first shoes were made in the early 1970s, the soles under the heel were heavily reinforced to make it possible to put the heels in front of the body to obtain a longer stride. Nothing can be more wrong than that. We've already mentioned that the fundamental form of running is for the foot to land under the body and push the runner upward and forward. To place the foot in front of the body and pull the body forward is a technique that the human body is not designed to perform. Each time you land on the heel, it slows down the forward movement unnecessarily, which is a big waste of energy because the body is biased. The consequences are not only that you are slowed down, but your risk of injury also increases.

Several running experts argue that modern running shoes have destroyed generations of runners. That might be going too far, but it's paradoxical that a product designed to protect and prevent injuries has destroyed the running technique and increased the propensity for injury for so many runners. To some extent structured shoes protect against the problems that occur when you land on the heel, but they can never replace a natural technique when it comes to running fast and avoiding injuries.

When one prevents a natural movement, other movements are negatively affected. If you land on your heels, you expose your body to an unnatural weight load. The bodyweight is received by the heels and is transferred to the knees, hips, and back. This is the main reason so many runners get loading injuries each year, especially in the knees and back. A recent study shows that heel-runners get twice as many injuries as front foot runners.

Landing on the front of the foot is part of a natural running style because your feet are built for it, and you not only get stronger feet but a more efficient running stride. When the ankle takes the entire bodyweight,

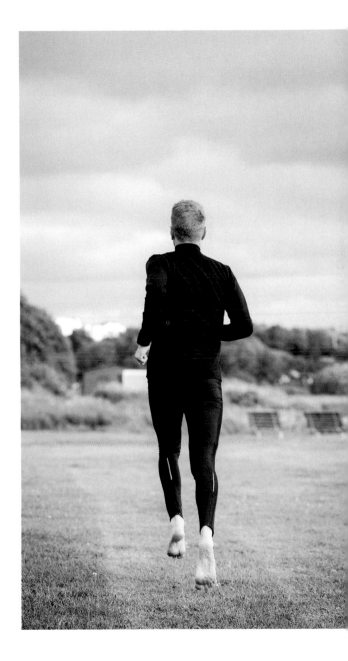

> **If you land on your heels, you expose your body to an unnatural weight load. The bodyweight is received by the heels and is transferred to the knees, hips, and back.**

it reduces the load on other joints that are put under stress from heel running.

Train barefoot sometimes

The criticism of running shoes has pioneered barefoot running. We've already discussed the huge advantages African runners get simply by running barefoot during their first years of running. What happens when you run without shoes is that you automatically land on the front part of the foot since there is no damper under the heels. The body instinctively adapts to a natural, more efficient running style where you rely on the built-in foot strength. An important part of this is that the pelvis automatically tilts slightly upward, which leads to the arch in the lower back decreasing so you have a better posture and can use your bodyweight to create

speed. You automatically get a much better running style when running without shoes—a stride similar to the one you had as a child.

Barefoot running is excellent training for those who want to learn better landing techniques and at the same time get stronger feet and calves. Right from the first stride without shoes, you'll feel how your feet are forced to work differently because you use muscles in the foot that remain completely passive when running with thick shoes. Another thing that happens when you land on the front part of the foot is that the ligaments and bones in the ankle joint are strengthened, which improves balance.

In elite sports, they have long been aware of the disadvantages of running shoess. Among jumpers and sprinters, where the load on the feet is significant, they practice a lot of barefoot techniques to strengthen their ankles. Lower intensity warm-up jogging and running is ideal to do without shoes even for long distance runners.

As barefoot running is strength training for the ankles, it's important to adjust gradually. If your body is accustomed to running shoes with two-centimeter-thick soles under the heel, it's a major change to run without shoes. This is partly because your foot muscles have been weakened by the shoes, and partly because it takes time to find your way back to a movement you haven't performed in twenty or thirty years.

The first barefoot workouts should be around 10 minutes of quiet running on soft surfaces, like grass or sand. If your feet or tendons don't get sore, increase the number of passes up to three times per week before adding a few minutes to the running distance. Understand that it may take several months before you can run 20–30 minutes in a row without any pain.

If you plan to run barefoot on asphalt, this will require a much longer adjustment period. The question is whether it's appropriate at all, given that our feet were not built to run on such hard surfaces. You sometimes see people on asphalt, running barefoot or with the so-called barefoot shoes that don't have soles. The hard surface is forcing them into a shortened stride with minimal knee lift and push-off, which means that they miss the point of barefoot running entirely—to run more naturally and with better running economy. Barefoot shoes work well on soft surfaces as

protection against sharp objects, but are not recommended for asphalt running.

Choose the right shoes

An alternative to running barefoot is to run with shoes that have thin and flexible soles, either proper racing shoes, or running shoes that don't have a thick heel cushion. Then, you get the best of both worlds—a shoe that is thin enough for you to be able to meet the ground in almost the same way as if you were running barefoot, and a sole that can be worn on harder surfaces. Just remember that, like with barefoot running, there will be a long adjustment period when you change to thinner shoes.

You should only run as long you manage to meet the ground with the front part of the foot. Otherwise the risk for injury is great because the shoes lack cushioning under the heel.

What determines if a shoe is good or bad for your running technique is the so-called "heel-toe drop", which indicates how thick the sole under the heel is compared to the footpad.

Since the 1970s, the standard for jogging shoes has been 12 millimeters. With such a thick sole under your heel, it's difficult to

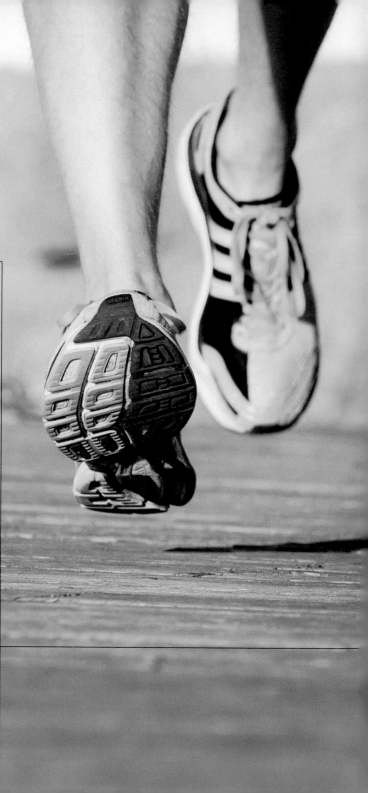

Flexibility makes your running energy-efficient

Several times, we've gone over how important the muscle's elastic energy is for endurance. A fourth of all energy consumed when running is "free" if you can only take advantage of the elasticity of the muscles.

Elite level runners are, of course, very good at this. Research shows, for example, that Kenyan runners have more elastic muscles than competitors from the Western world. This means that their leg muscles are better at extracting energy in the landing of each stride. But you can also get better at lightening the force against the ground that occurs when you land. That way, you can recycle a large part of the consumed energy, and that makes your running more energy efficient. Physiologists call the muscles' ability to recycle energy the stretch-shortening cycle. The name comes from the fact that the muscle is first stretched out (stretch) before it shrinks to develop force (shortening). This continuous flow has also given its name to the so-called running cycle (see the spread on pages 92–93), which includes four phases of the running stride.

In each phase some muscles are working to develop the force that is used both for the run and to charge energy in other resting muscles. In the next phase, the roles are reversed, and the muscles continue to switch between working and recharging over and over again.

The stretch-shortening cycle is the basis for understanding how running works. The point is that the elastic force doesn't cost any energy in the form of extra oxygen because it's created by itself through the running stride. The more you can use muscle elasticity as a power source, the lower the oxygen consumption will be and the faster you can run. In recent years there have been numerous research papers on the stretch-shortening cycle's impact on long distance running. Besides the energy recycling, the elasticity of the muscles contributes to

- reduced accumulation of waste products in the blood
- lower body temperature during exercise
- reduced fatigue in the thighs and calves.

In addition, the elastic energy gives a tension in the muscle that makes the power development faster. It is very important for the running economy; among other things, is reduces the contact time with the ground during each foot landing, especially if the Achilles tendon and muscles in the arch of the foot are tensed right before they are about to work. One of the drawbacks of running in shoes with thick cushioning is that the foot cannot feel the contact with the ground, and therefore a tension is not created in either the ankle, legs, or trunk.

In order to be able to take advantage of the elastic energy, you'll need an efficient running technique with a step that is relaxed and large enough so the muscles stretch out and can be charged with energy before they are put to work again. You can also improve your elastic capacity with jump and strength exercises. In jump exercises, the muscles practice slowing down the force of the landing, which improves the rebound effect—i.e. the muscle elasticity. You get a shorter contact time with the ground and save energy compared to if you collapse in a slow landing. This is much like the difference between how a well-pumped ball and a deflated ball meet the ground.

Jump training gives you an increased elastic muscular power without increased energy expenditure, which means your running economy improves. Several studies show that regular jump exercising improves running time by an average of 3 percent in just a few weeks. This means a cut of about a minute on a 5 kilometer run can be achieved by jump training alone.

land on the front part of the foot and the chances are that you will instead roll your heel. Racing shoes and shoes with thinner soles, on the other hand, have a heel-toe drop of 0–8 millimeters. The lower the heel, the harder it is to land on the heel, which forces your feet to meet the ground more actively and with a shorter period of contact. As a result, the foot lands more under the body, and the pelvis is slightly tilted upward and pushed forward, and you have a better posture just like when you run barefoot.

Thanks to better running technique, running economy is improved by almost 6 percent when switching from regular running shoes to running barefoot. The effect, which corresponds to 15–20 minutes in a marathon, is most likely the same in switching to shoes with thin soles.

Your stride should be long . . . and high

A question that often comes up is whether one should strive for a short or long running stride. The correct answer is neither. The stride length is actually a result of your running technique and not something you should consciously try to change.

Comparisons show that elite runners have longer steps than those who run for exercise, while the stride rhythm is the same—180 to 200 steps per minute. The elite runner's longer stride is mainly due to better technique, with the hips in a more forward position to take advantage of the push-off force and the falling reflex.

In order for a longer running stride to be advantageous, it must contribute to a better running economy. If you extend the stride by putting the foot forward and landing on the heel, the step becomes longer but at the cost of making the movement slower and consuming much more energy. Concentrate instead on working from the hips, so that your running stride lengthens naturally and efficiently. Using the test described on page 156, you can measure how your stride length develops.

It makes sense that a long running stride would be beneficial. Equally obvious is it that up and down movements waste energy because the force should be directed forward. Right?

Nope. Take a look at Haile Gebrselassie or any other international elite runner and you'll see that this is not true. At every step, they lift their knees considerably higher than the average exercise runner. The reason this is good for running economy is because of gravity.

To understand how gravitational force affects your running, imagine that you're holding a heavy iron ball in your hand. If you want to throw the ball far away, then you must target the force of your throw upward. If you throw it straight forward, then the ball will be pulled down to the ground right from the beginning. The force of gravity affects your body in the same way. Like the iron ball, you have to direct the force by running diagonally upward and forward. Studies of elite runners show that their push-off force is directed considerably more upward than forward by controlling their muscle power upward and adapting to the laws of gravity rather than fighting against them. But where does the force that propels the runners forward come from? This is where the falling reflex comes into play. If you run with your hips tilted upward, then the combination of gravity, push-off force, and the falling reflex becomes a forward motion that lifts you up just enough to give a long running stride with low energy consumption. But the feet, knees, and hips are working vertically. The body's center of gravity should, however, move as little as possible vertically, and elite runners' hips stay leveled from start to finish. The hips' movement pushes the body's center of gravity forward, but does not affect it vertically.

THE RUNNING CYCLE

The running stride is a continuous movement that is divided into landing, push-off, forward-, and backward swing of the leg. The stride becomes the most effective when you run

» in a position where you use your bodyweight to push forward

» in a way so that the muscles are pulled apart to develop the maximum amount of elastic force.

1. LANDING

The right leg lands underneath the body to minimize contact with the ground, while the extension muscles in the foot, leg, and trunk curb the force that brings you to the ground to keep the body's center of gravity in an elevated position. Since the landing is done on the front of the sole of the foot, the elastic muscles under the foot pull apart while the Achilles tendon is stretched out by gravity. The efforts to curb the force that bring you down to the ground store energy in the foot, Achilles tendon, and muscles of the front thigh, the buttocks, and the trunk. By landing underneath the body you also create a falling reflex that makes the hips push the motion forward.

2. PUSH-OFF

A few milliseconds later, the energy that has been stored in the landing is used in the push-off. The power goes in a straight line from the foot to the upward-facing hips and presses your body upward and forward. The ankle, leg, and buttocks are stretched to build maximum power. The upright upper body makes the hips angle upward, which makes the muscles in the stomach and hip flexors on the front of the thigh pull apart and get charged with energy. Thanks to the forward tilted hip position your bodyweight creates a force that moves you forward.

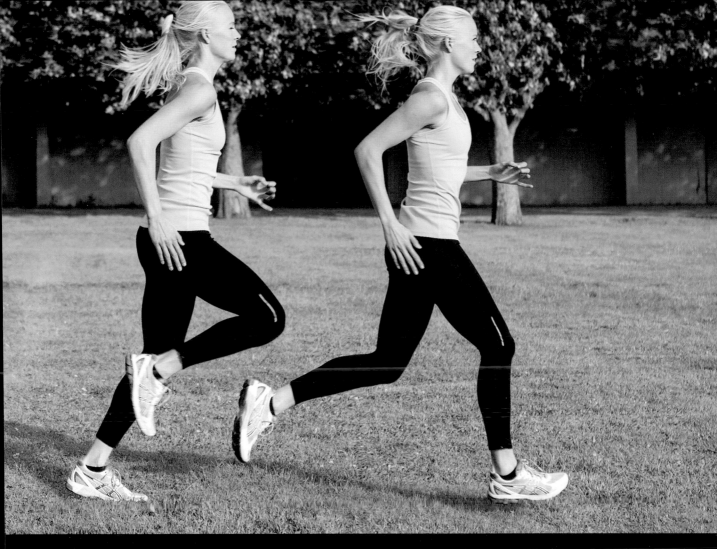

3. FORWARD LEG STRIDE

When the leg extends forward, the hip flexors and the abdominal muscles have both been charged with energy in the previous phase to make the movement as quick and efficient as possible. Now in the forward stride, it's the muscles of the back thigh and buttocks that stretch out in the sequence to work optimally. The leg is striding forward with a pointed knee to meet the falling reflex that is created when the second leg lands

4. BACKWARD LEG STRIDE

The back thigh muscles and buttocks pull the leg back, and thanks to the elastic energy, the stride becomes more powerful so that the foot lands under the body in the next phase. The power in the backward leg stride is reinforced by angling that leg's hip downward and back. Since both hips move in tandem, the other hip angles upward and forward, which empowers the forward stride of the other leg.

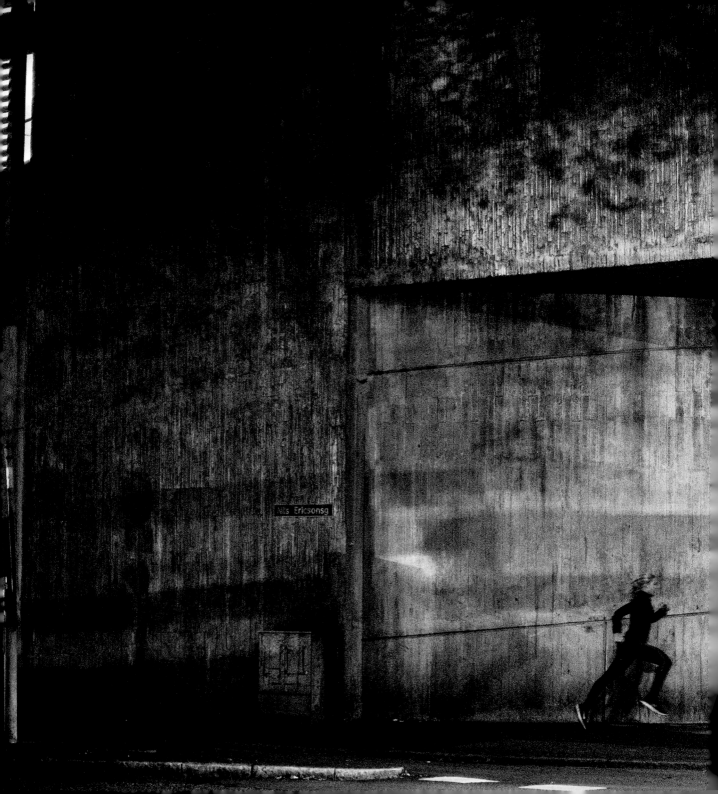

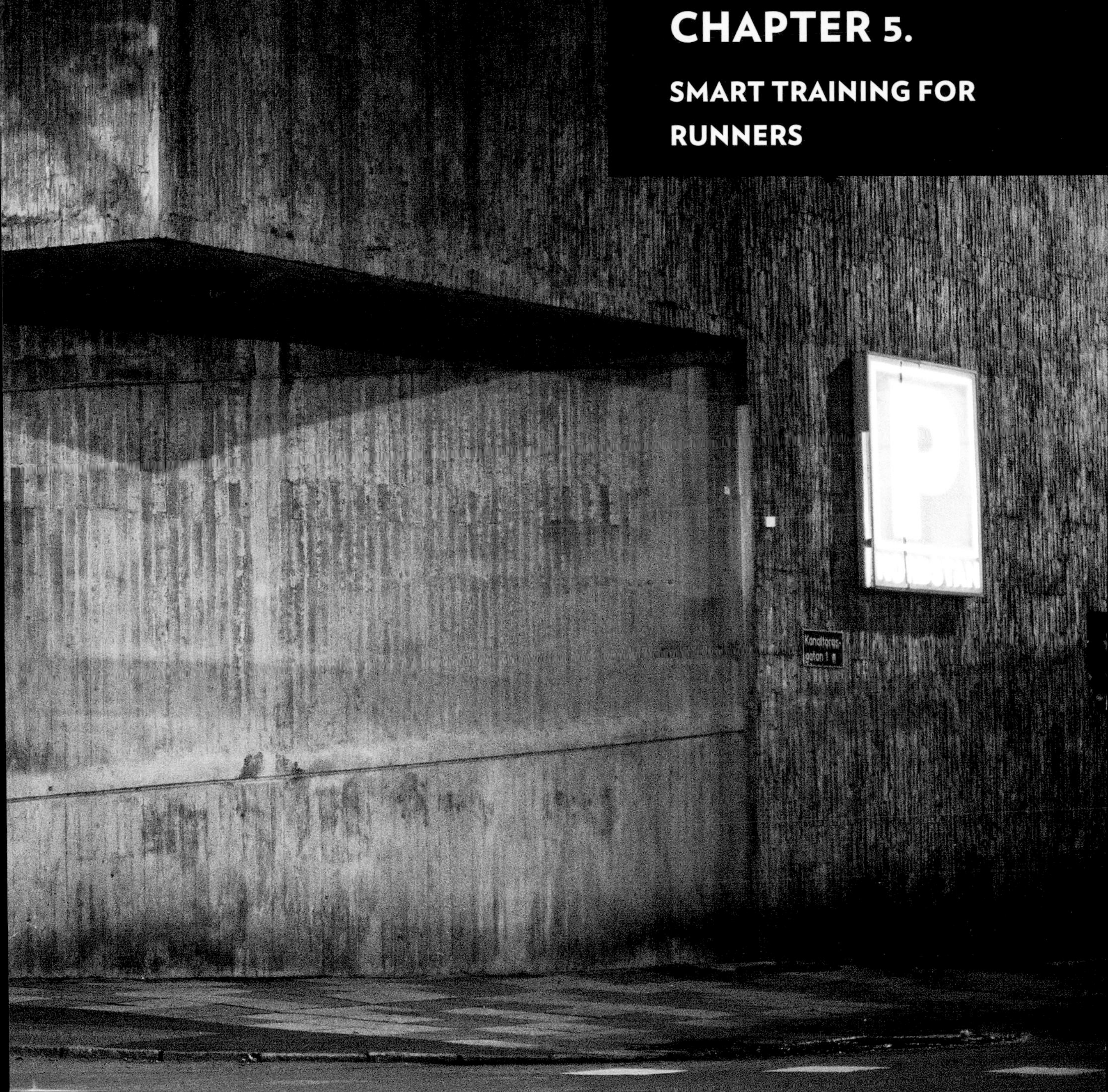

5.

YOU'VE REACHED THE BOOK'S PRACTICAL SECTION, WHERE THE FOCUS IS ON THE THREE TECHNIQUE CHAPTERS.

» Hips (Chapter 6)

» Shoulders (Chapter 7)

» Foot landing (Chapter 8)

Most people should probably begin by training hip work, but if you have very stiff shoulders or run with a curved back you should probably start with Chapter 7 instead. If you're already running with your body at a straight line and your hips in the correct position, then you can start by focusing on your foot landing. Perform the exercises in the chapter you have selected and gradually increase the degree of difficulty. There are also practical suggestions for technique workouts to help you get started. But in order to run more efficiently, you need to train more than your running technique, and therefore each chapter contains strength and flexibility exercises that specifically focus on the hips, shoulders, or feet.

When you start to learn a new running stride, you should prioritize technical training, but it is, of course, good to train your overall physique. In Chapter 9, there's a strength program for runners of all levels. In the same chapter you'll also find exercises to train muscle flexibility.

Jumping exercises to improve your foot landing can be found in Chapter 8. However, as jump training also improves the leg muscles' elasticity, if you're focusing on hip or shoulder training, you can add these exercises to your strength training. Just remember to read the instructions carefully.

The book's tenth and final chapter contains four tests that will give you feedback on how your running economy and technique have developed.

How to practice your technique

1. Learn the new movement
2. Practice it in your running
3. Control the movement at high speed

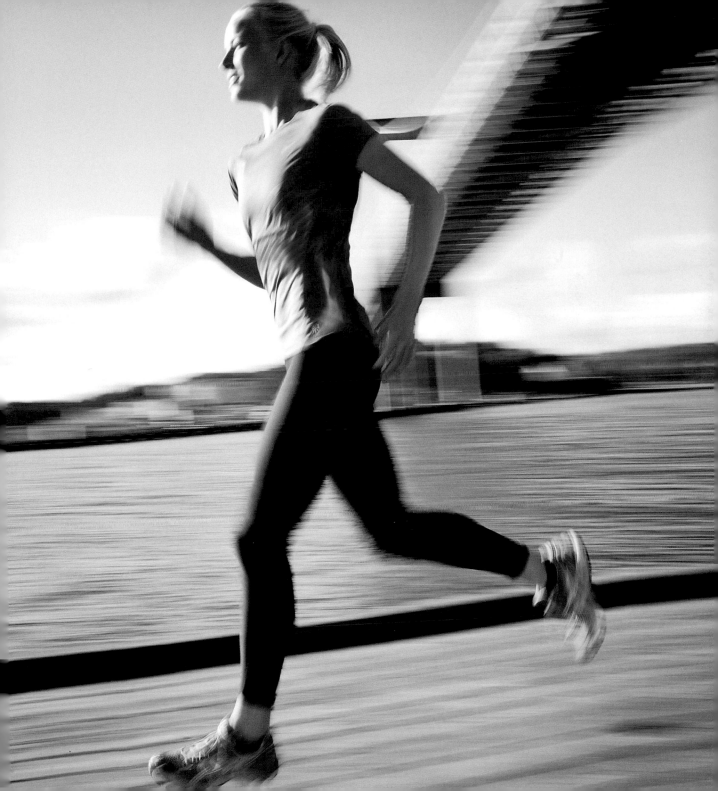

The technique programs start with standing and walking exercises, which you can do at home, in the apartment, or in the garden. This means that you can easily practice your technique several times a week, maybe even every day, and you'll learn to do it properly faster. Try to practice at least twice a week for about 15 minutes—any longer than that is difficult because the brain quickly tires of concentrating on doing it right.

Remember to put your focus on doing the exercises as accurately as possible, not on keeping a fast pace. It helps if you're well rested both mentally and physically, and it's best if you practice your techniques before your regular run. This will make it easier to transfer the movements to your normal running stride. Just remember to first jog lightly for 5–10 minutes to warm up your muscles.

In most of the exercises, you work with a much larger range of motion than you should have when you run. You lift the knee higher, push through the hips more, and have a larger arm swing. The point in exaggerating the motions in your technical training is that it improves the learning; you will more quickly learn to use your hips, while gaining increased mobility and reducing the risk of injury.

As soon as you learn the correct position, try using it in the run. In the beginning, you may run slower in order to concentrate on your running stride, but once your muscles get used to the new technique, you can increase the pace. When you do it right you will notice it becomes easier to run, and the stride feels softer and more powerful because the muscles and joints are working more naturally.

Eventually, the movements become automatic and then you only need to think about technique at the beginning of the run and check it regularly. How often depends on how deep your technique has been ingrained and how intense the run is.

When to switch the focus of your technique

You decide yourself how long you should focus on each technical element. Do not stop too early; do not expect that you will run more efficiently after only a week. You will probably begin to discover the progress after a few weeks of training. At that point you'll only be at the beginning of a long-term change, and therefore it will definitely be worth it to continue for a while longer. Take the tests in Chapter 10 to determine your development, and if nothing happens after a few weeks of ambitious training, you may need to go back to the first exercises and find out where you lost the thread.

For some runners, it may be smartest to never change the focus area. This is partly because it will simultaneously affect the rest of the running stride if you get really good at running with the hips or shoulders in the right position, and partly because you risk losing what you're learning if you change your focus too soon. Of course, you could try to change afterward, but don't be surprised if you benefit in the long-term by sticking with one element of the technique.

If you're an elite runner and already have a good running technique, then you will probably gain the most by switching between the various technical elements. The program contains exercises that can be done with more precision to make your running technique and your ability to run more economical, and there is always room from improvement even if you've already come a long way.

Keep in mind

» *Do it accurately*
It's only when you perform a movement the right way that you strengthen the interaction between the brain and the muscles. Therefore it's better to do an exercise a few times accurately than to do many reps improperly.

» *Alternate the training*
Take advantage of as many exercises in the program as you can handle. Varying the challenges stimulates your brain, and in this way, strengthens the connections with the muscles and allows you to quickly learn a new movement—provided that you do it accurately.

» *Let your trigger help you*
Create a mental image of the perfect motion that you're striving for. The picture should be clear so you can use it as a trigger—a body-altering thought of moving accurately when you run.

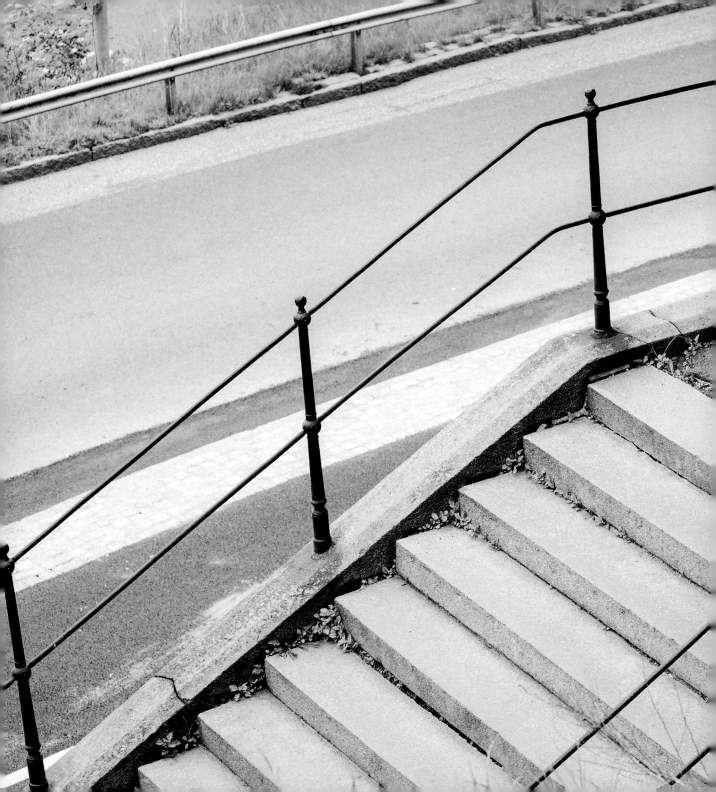

CHAPTER 6.

THE HIPS—THE ENGINE OF THE RUNNING STRIDE

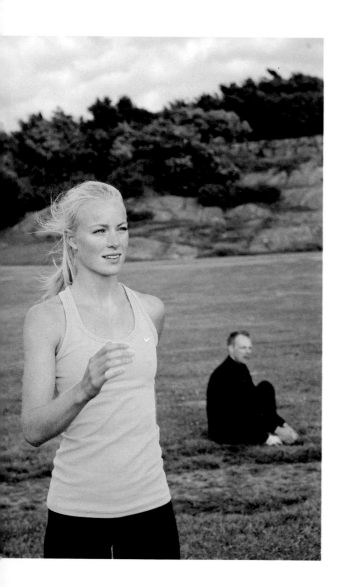

6.

THE HIPS ARE THE ENGINE OF YOUR RUNNING STRIDE. IT'S THE HIPS THAT PUSH THE RUN FORWARD SO THAT YOU CAN TAKE ADVANTAGE OF YOUR OWN BODYWEIGHT TO CREATE FORWARD MOTION.

Hip work in running is all about three elements—tilt the pelvis upward, press the hips forward, and bring out the hips' sideways mobility. It may sound complicated to do all that when you run, but since all three are natural movements, the last two come automatically if you learn how to tilt the hips.

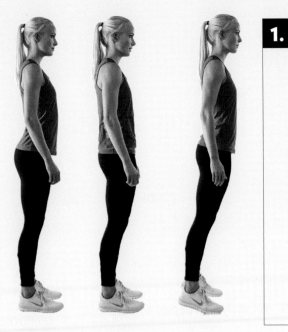

1.

Angle the hips upward and push them forward: Stand with your feet shoulder width apart. Then tilt the pelvis upward and flatten the arch of the lower back by tightening the muscles in the buttocks and lower abdomen. Hold for 2–3 seconds and switch between positions 1 and 2 a few times. Then go from position 2 to 3 by pushing the hips until your heels are lifted from the ground so that you're almost about to fall forward. The hips and torso should create a straight line; don't cheat by simply leaning your chest forward. This is the basic position in running that you should always start from. Hold for a few seconds in position 3 and repeat as often as possible.

2.

Walk or run in place: Stand in position 2 above. Lift your knees and land on the front part of the foot under the body without moving forward. Swing the arms. The feeling of how you land under the body is the foundation of how to use the hips accurately in running. Do 2–3 x 30 seconds.

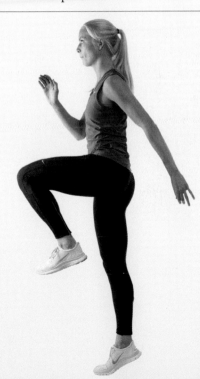

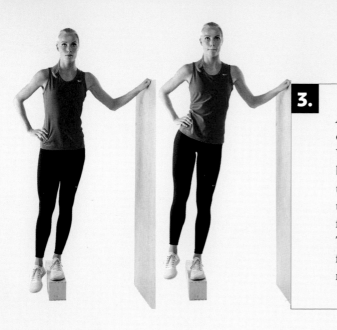

3.

Move the hips sideways: Stand on a step on one leg with your other foot in the air. You can also stand on a flat surface if you bend the other leg slightly so that it doesn't touch the ground. Lift the hip of the leg that is in the air and make circles upward-forward-down-backwards with the hip. This exercise trains the hip's ability to follow the leg in the forward stride. Do 10 repetitions per leg.

4.

Walk like a power walker: Use the movement from exercise 3 and walk with exaggerated side movements in your hips. Feel the stride start from the hip rather than from the thigh and notice how each hip extends each stride forward. Remember that the hip should be higher on the side where the leg strides forward. Walk 2–3 x 30 meters.

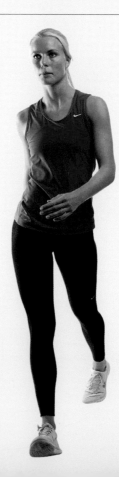

5. *Lying down knee lift with active hips:* Lie straight and avoid arching your lower back by tilting the hips as in exercise 1. Place one hand under the arch of your back to make sure it is flat. Now keep the hip position while lifting one knee and feel how the same side of the hip elevates. Feel how the muscles in the buttocks squeeze on the other side of the hip. Hold for 2–3 seconds and repeat 5 times for each leg.

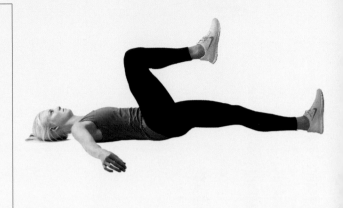

6. *Standing knee lift with active hips:* Stand roughly 3 feet from a wall and support yourself against it. Lift the knee up and forward and let the hip on that side follow. You shouldn't just lift the knee but feel how the pressure against the arms increases when the hip pulls the entire weight of the body forward. Do 5 repetitions for each leg, one leg at a time.

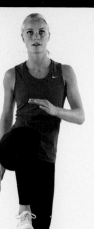

7.

Hip walk: Start by walking in place as in exercise 2. Then angle the hips upward and push them forward so that you fall forward and start to walk. Feel how your own bodyweight pushes you forward through the hips and that the feet help create the right feeling by landing under the body. Walk 2–3 x 20 meters.

8.

Knee lift running/skipping: Run in place as in exercise 2 with high knees and land with your feet under your body. Press your hips forward as in exercise 7 and start running with high knees pointing forward. Remember to land with stretched legs under the body so that your hips push you forward. Run 2–3 x 20–30 meters.

9.

Towing with a thick elastic band or rope (that does not scrape against you): Overcome resistance by landing with your foot under you so that your bodyweight pushes you forward with your hips in a forward position. The resistance should be heavy enough that you have to use your body weight by pushing your hips forward (to power ahead). Run 3–5 x 20–30 meters. Between each run you can run relaxedly for 50 meters without the load, try to push yourself forward in the same way with the hips.

10.

Running uphill: Run up a low incline with the same emphasis on putting the foot under the body, and push yourself forward with the hip in a forward position. Run 3–5 x 30–60 meters.

11.

Coordination run: Start from the knee lift run (exercise 8) at a slow pace so you land with the feet under the body and allow your hips to push forward. Increase the speed gradually by pressing the hips even more, and increase the sense of falling in every stride. Emphasize technique rather than speed. Run 100 meters 3–5 times.

12.

Short sit-ups for the inner transversus abdominis muscle: The lower back should always be touching the ground. Go down slowly so you work in the muscle's eccentric phase. Do the exercise either as part of your technique training without getting tired, or as strength training—in that case, do at least 20 repetitions x 3.

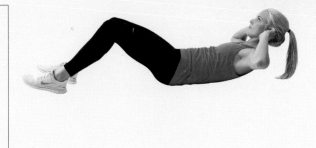

13.

Plank: A static exercise where you tense the abdominals and buttocks to get a perfectly straight body and to flatten the lower back. Stop the exercise when you can no longer remain in a straight position. Do it 2–3 times for about 1 minute.

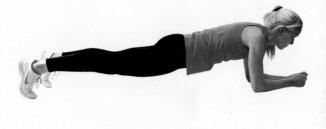

14.

Reclined hip and leg lifts: Lift the hips and one leg by pushing off with the foot on the other leg. Avoid touching your butt to the ground on the way down. Do 2–3 x 10 per leg.

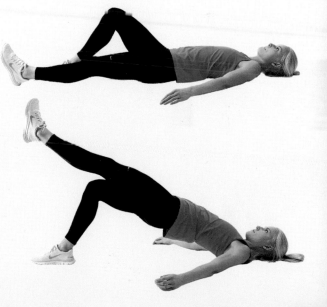

Stretching exercises are important for hip mobility. To warm up, do exercises 15–16, and do stretches in exercises 17–19 after the session so that the stiffened muscles can regain their length. Hold the extended position for 20–30 seconds.

15.

Leg swings with a straight leg: Work with a long and soft movement where you stretch the ankles on the grounded leg in the extended position. Remember to keep the upper body straight and feel the hip move with the swinging leg. Repeat ten times back and forth with each leg.

16.

Sideways leg swings: The same emphases as exercise 15. Repeat ten times outward and inward with each leg.

17.

Hip flexors: To access the muscle, angle the hip upward and straighten the arch of the lower back. Gently press the lower part of the pelvis forward.

18.

The hamstring muscles on the back of the thighs: Here, you arch instead and bend the knee lightly. Push yourself forward from the navel, not your chest, or you'll miss the effect of the stretch and load the back incorrectly.

19.

The buttocks: Pull the knee inward with your arm to access the muscle.

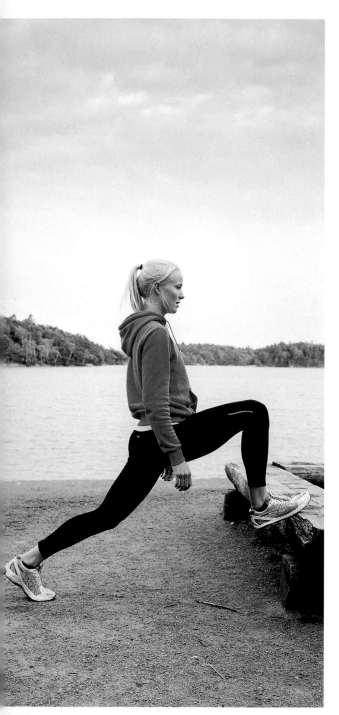

Get started!

The training is planned so that you first learn what it feels like to perform the hip movements: tilting the pelvis upward, pushing the hip forward and moving it sideways. After that, you can practice letting your hip propel you forward in the run at the same time as your feet land under the body. Once you find the sense of falling, you should try to control it in motion, from slow technique exercises to running at full speed.

Exercises 1, 2, and 7 are the most important. In exercise 1, you'll learn the basic positions for running. The 2nd gives you the right feeling for landing under the hip. Exercise 7 is to combine the hip position and the foot landing to find the sense of falling.

Remember that it's better to do fewer repetitions with proper technique than to rush through the entire program. The first few times you might only manage to do one or two exercises properly, but if you're careful, you'll get better the more you practice.

Three technique sessions

If you don't want to put together your own training programs, it's perfectly fine to do these three sessions. Be prepared that you may have to train level 1 dozens of times before you're ready to move on. If level 2 feels too tough, you can either go back to level 1 and improve there or do the new exercises very slowly and maybe ask someone to film you.

THREE TECHNIQUE SESSIONS FOR THE HIPS

LEVEL 1 – FIND THE HIPS' CORRECT POSITION

» Focus on technique exercises 1–6 and be particularly careful with 1–2

» Warm up with mobility exercises 15–16 before your session

» Do exercises 17–19 to stretch after each session

» Do the strength exercises 13–15 regularly

LEVEL 2 – FEEL THE HIP PUSHING YOU FORWARD

» Focus on transferring what you learned from exercise 1–2 to exercise 7

» Try exercises 8–11 to practice the sense of falling

» Be careful with mobility and strength exercises

» Do test B in Chapter 10 to see if your stride length has changed

LEVEL 3 – LET THE HIP PUSH YOU FORWARD IN YOUR REGULAR RUNNING

» Warm up with one or more of exercises 7–11 to help you find the sense of how your hip pushes you forward and your feet land under the body

» When you run, feel how you use your own bodyweight to power forward, possibly with the help of a trigger from the exercises

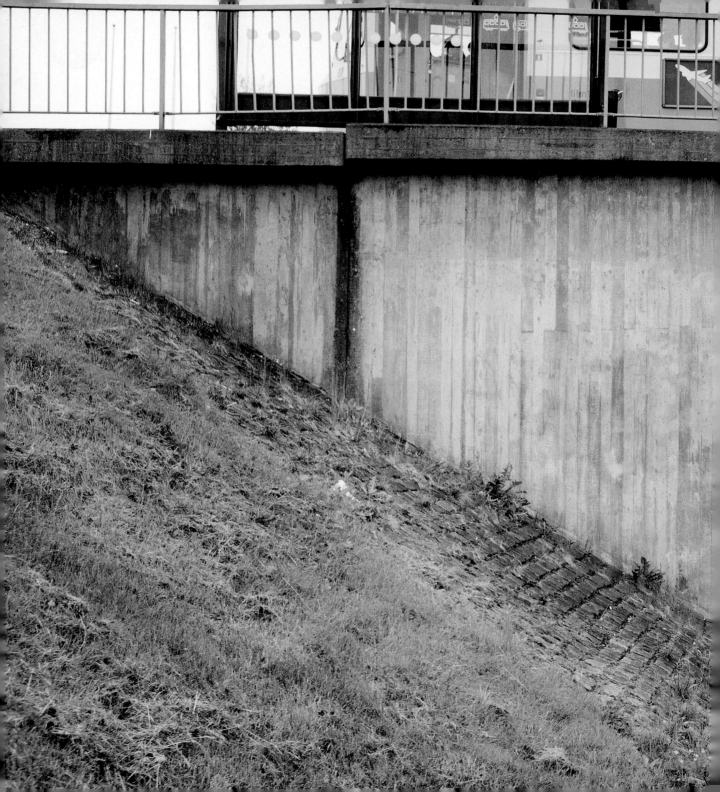

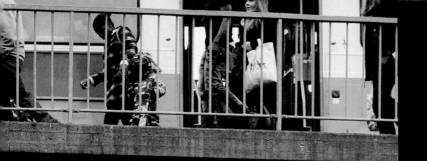

CHAPTER 7.

SHOULDERS— PROPER POSTURE

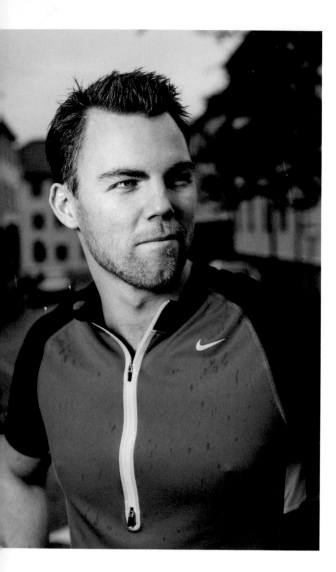

STIFF SHOULDERS ARE THE BIGGEST ENERGY THIEF IN RUNNING. THE IDEAL IS TO RUN WITH LOW AND RELAXED SHOULDERS. THIS GIVES YOU BETTER POSTURE, A LARGER ARM SWING, AND MORE POWER IN YOUR RUNNING STRIDE.

Tension in the shoulder joint is almost always related to a slightly forward bent posture, which is caused by poor mobility in the shoulder and chest muscles while having weak muscles in the upper back. To cure tense shoulders, strengthen the back muscles around the shoulder blades and simultaneously increase the mobility in the shoulders and chest muscles. Then you not only become a better runner but get a better-looking posture as well.

Tip! Remember to relax your stomach when you're working the shoulders, neck, and chest muscles. Tensed abdominal muscles counteract the stretching of the upper back. When you practice your posture, you should also remember to strive to have low shoulders while lifting the ribs.

1.

Stretch the chest muscles: Stand with your right leg slightly bent in front of you and your left leg pointed out. Place your right elbow against a wall just above shoulder height; feel the weight of the body resting on the right heel so that you are not hanging on your arm. Tilt your upper body forward and inward so that it extends into the right chest muscle and smoothly increases the pressure on each exhalation. Do 10 breaths per side x 2.

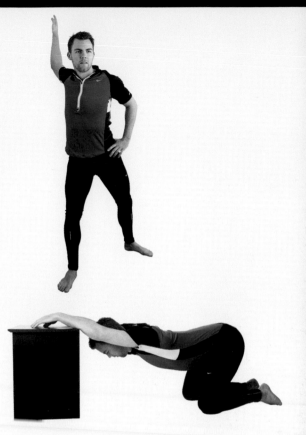

2.

Stretch shoulders, chest, and back: Crouch on your knees, slightly wider than hip width apart and arch your back. Feel how you distribute the body weight evenly on both legs and upper body. Rest your arms on a chair or a table. Let your upper body "fall" between your arms so that you stretch your chest, shoulders, and mid-back. Relax and sink deeper on each exhale. Make 10 breaths x 2.

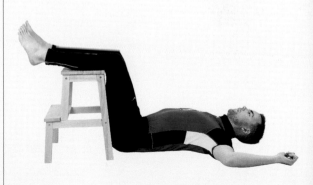

3.

Strengthen the shoulders and shoulder blades: Improves strength for the shoulder blades and increase mobility in the shoulders. Lie as shown in the photo with low shoulders and with your chin tucked in. Press your hands against the floor so that you feel the back of your shoulders and shoulder blades tighten. Remember to keep your arms pointing out with palms facing up. Do 3 x 10 repetitions of 1–2 seconds.

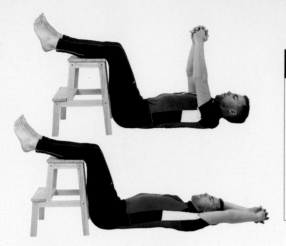

4.

Shoulder stretch: Lie as shown in the photo with straight arms and clasped hands. Slowly lower your arms as you inhale and lift them as you exhale. In the lower position you practice the mobility of the shoulders, going as far down as you can without forcing, without bending your arms, and remembering to keep low shoulders. Do 10 repetitions x 3.

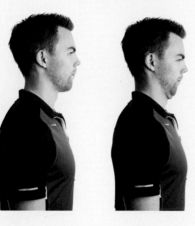

5.

Strengthen the neck: Start with a neutral upright position and then pull your head back so you get a double chin and feel your neck stretching. Do 10 repetitions x 3.

6.

Back extension with active shoulder blades: Lie on your stomach with your legs together, lift your back slightly and stretch your arms upward with the thumbs up. Then pull your arms backwards and upwards as shown in the photo. Feel that you are working the back of the shoulders and between the shoulder blades. From the most extended position go back to the forward position and then lower the upper body and arms to the floor. Rest for 1 second and start over. Do 5–10 repetitions x 3.

7.

Arm circles: Sit down as shown in the photo, stretch your arms out straight to just under shoulder height, with bent fingers, palms facing down, and thumbs pointing forward. Arch, lower your shoulders, squeeze your shoulder blades together, and make small circles with your arms upward-forward-downward. Then, turn your arms in a half circle with your thumbs pointing back and do circles the other way, upward-backward-downward. If you do not feel any tension around the shoulder blades, then try to hold your arms a little further back. Make 30 circles forward and 30 circles backward x 3.

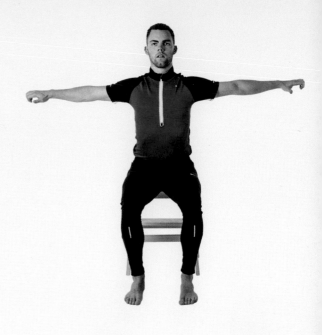

8.

Stretching the neck muscles: Sit down, bend your head to the side and hold the shoulder down on the opposite side. The shoulder should be as far away as possible from the ear on the other side. Feel how it stretches the neck. After 20–30 seconds tilt your head slightly forward to access the other neck muscle. Now, it stretches a little further down around the shoulder blades. Stay for 20–30 seconds in this position and then change sides.

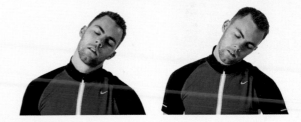

9.

Mobility of the back: Arch to the maximum for 5 seconds, then round up the back for 5 seconds. Repeat x 5 in each position.

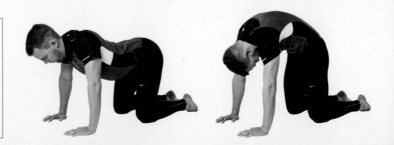

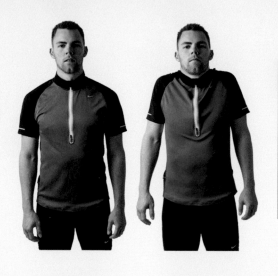

10.

The shoulders' movement upwards–downwards: Pull your shoulders up towards your ears as far as you can before you let them down and relax. Feel the difference between the high, tense shoulders, and relaxed position with low shoulders. Hold for 2–3 seconds in both positions x 10.

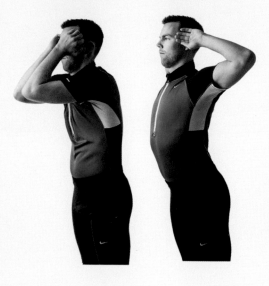

11.

The shoulders' movement forward–backward: Lift the elbows forward as shown in the picture so they meet in a line with your throat, then drag them out backward, and let the shoulders follow back, so your chest is broad and you feel a tension in your shoulder blades. Try to keep low shoulders throughout the movement. Hold for 2–3 seconds in each position x 10.

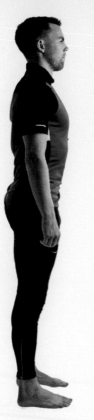

12.

Vertical line: Stand with your arms at your sides. Relax your shoulders and pull them gently downward towards your back. Strengthen the movement by making yourself broader across the chest and feel how the back stretches when you raise your ribs. Feel how your neck is stretched to form the top link in a straight vertical line from the ears down to the ankles. Remember to tilt your hips upwards so they are also in the straight line. Try to stay relaxed in this position for 30 seconds x 3–5.

13.

Arm swing: Use the same position as in exercise 12. Swing your arms in a relaxed manner and feel how the movement becomes easy and automatic when the shoulders are low and towards the back. Try to bring this feeling to your running. Swing for 10–15 seconds x 2–3.

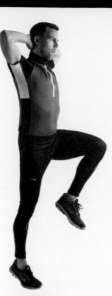

14.

Walk with upright posture: Start from the vertical position, then walk forward with your hands resting on your neck. Remember to be broad across the chest and have low shoulders. Avoid compensating posture by arching. Walk 20 meters x 2–3.

15.

Smooth jumps: Jump on one leg twice then switch to the other leg (right-right-left-left) with the same emphasis as in exercise 14. Jump 30 meters x 2–3.

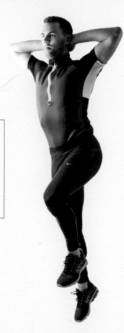

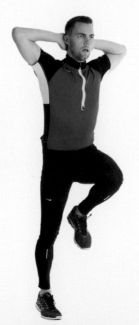

16.

High knees: Knee lift running with hands behind the head. The body is vertical and the hips are tilted upward and in a forward position. Do 2–3 x 20–30 meters.

17.

Coordination run: Run slowly with a vertical body, shoulders relaxed, and your hands behind your head. Increase the pace gradually and drop your arms after 30–50 meters and continue to run. Try to maintain the low shoulders and the power in the stride by following the leg motion gently with your arms. Run about 100 meters 3–5 times.

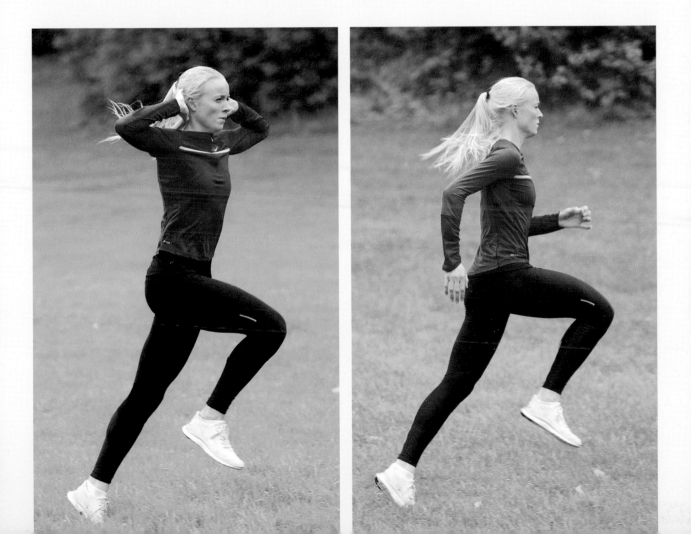

Get started!

Start with the strength and mobility program and also practice your posture, from standing and walking to eventually running with a more upright torso. If you have stiff shoulders, then you probably need to train strength and mobility for a long period. Make it a habit to work through all or part of the strength and mobility program at least three times every week.

If you're exercising ambitiously, then you'll soon find the correct position with low, relaxed shoulders. Try to run that way, and you'll discover that your arm swing is getting longer, and because of that, the running stride lengthens, which substantially improves your running economy.

Remember that it's better to do fewer repetitions with proper technique than to rush through an entire program. The first few times you may only manage to do one or two exercises, but if you're careful, you'll get better the more you practice.

Three technique sessions

If you don't want to put together your own exercise program, then do these three sessions. Be prepared that you may have to train level 1 dozens of times before you're ready to move on. If level 2 feels too tough, then you can either go back to level 1 and become even better there, or do the new exercises very slowly and maybe ask someone to film you.

THREE TECHNIQUE SESSIONS FOR THE SHOULDERS

LEVEL 1 – FIND YOUR VERTICAL POSTURE

» Do the flexibility and strength exercises 1–9 as often as you can so you get back the mobility in your shoulders, preferably three times per week

» Do posture exercises 10–12

» Do posture exercise 13 when you have low shoulders

» Try to walk with low, relaxed shoulders and feel the difference

LEVEL 2 – MOVE WITH LOW SHOULDERS AND A VERTICAL POSTURE

» Do flexibility and strength exercises 1–9 to maintain or improve mobility in the shoulders

» Do posture exercise 12 to practice the vertical posture

» Do technique exercises 14–16 to practice having upright posture in motion

» Do technique exercise 17 to feel how important the arm swing is

LEVEL 3 – RUN WITH LOW SHOULDERS AND UPRIGHT UPPER BODY

» Do flexibility and strength exercises 1–9 to maintain or improve mobility in the shoulders

» Choose from exercises 14–17 to empower the sense of an upright posture and a "free" arm swing

» Use that feeling later in your running

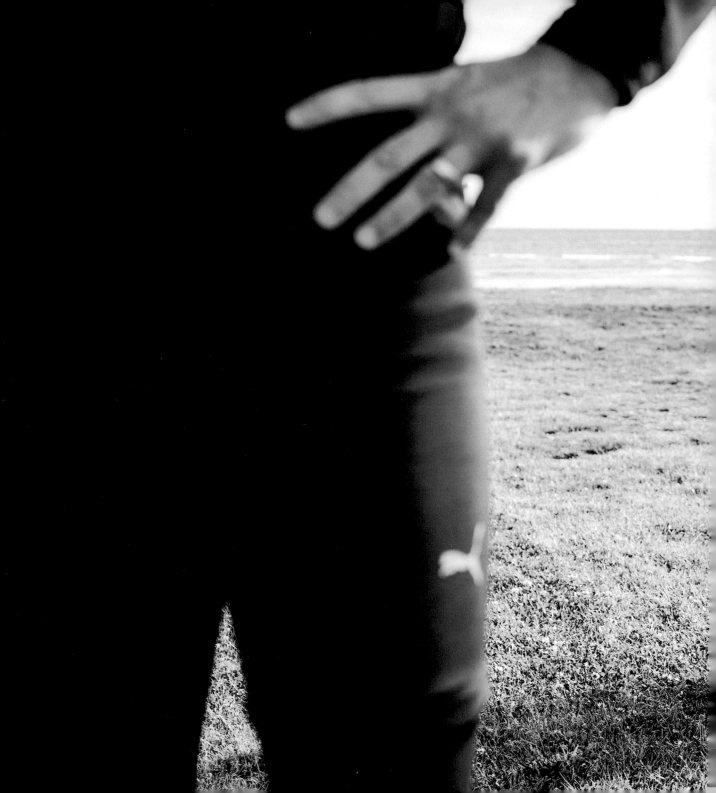

CHAPTER 8.

THE FEET—
FIND THE RIGHT
FOOT LANDING

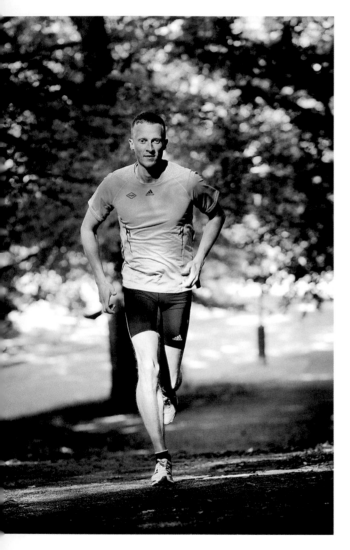

8.

**WHEN YOU LAND FURTHER FOR-
WARD ON YOUR FOOT WHILE KEEP-
ING IT UNDERNEATH THE BODY, YOU
RUN FASTER AND REDUCE THE RISK
OF DAMAGING YOUR KNEES, HIPS,
AND BACK. TO COPE WITH SUCH A
FOOT LANDING, TWO THINGS ARE
REQUIRED: YOU MUST RUN WITH
YOUR BODY IN THE RIGHT POSITION
AND YOUR ANKLE MUSCLES MUST BE
STRONG ENOUGH.**

Foot training differs from hip and
shoulder training in that it builds on
what you have already learned when
running with your hips in the forward
position. If you haven't done that ho-
mework, then it's better to practice
the exercises in Chapter 6.

1.

Toe walk: Walk with stretched ankles. Try to get as elevated as possible. Walk 20 meters x 2.

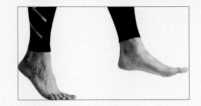

2.

Heel walk: Walk on your heels so that your toes point up and avoid bending at the hip. Walk 20 meters x 2.

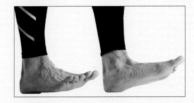

3.

Rotate the foot inward/outward: Turn your foot inward (supination) and outward (pronation), hold for 2–3 seconds in the extended position. Repeat 20 x 2 on each foot.

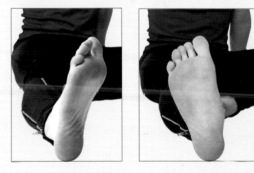

4.

Pinch and spread your toes: Enlarge the movements in the extended position and hold for 2–3 seconds. Repeat 20 x 2 on each foot.

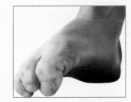
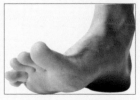

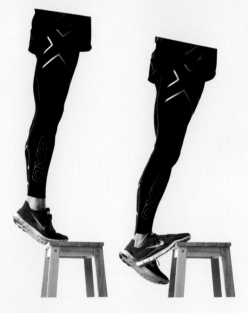
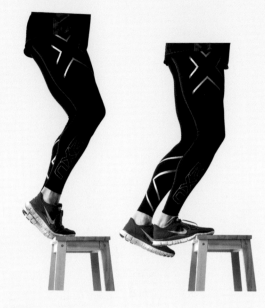

5. *Heel raises with straight legs:* Stand with the front part of your feet on a step, a board, or something similar to enhance your range of motion. Push yourself as high up you can using both your feet, and lower yourself slowly down on one leg at a time to get eccentric training in the outer calf muscle. Do 15 repetitions per leg x 2–3.

6. *Heel raises with bent knees:* Work the same way as in exercise 5 but with the knees slightly bent throughout the movement to instead train the deep calf muscle. Do 15 repetitions per leg x 2–3.

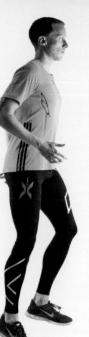

7. *Rebound jumps on one leg:* Perform fast and short vertical jumps, landing high up on the foot. Jump 30 seconds per leg x 3.

8. *Stretching the outer calf muscle:* Press the hips forward and let the back heel remain on the ground.

9. *Stretching the inner calf muscle:* This is the same as the previous exercise, but with bent knee. You should feel a stretch a little further down toward the Achilles tendon. Press the knee forward and keep the back heel on the ground.

10.

Walk or run in place: Get used to landing with the front part of the foot underneath the body. Do 30 seconds x 2–3.

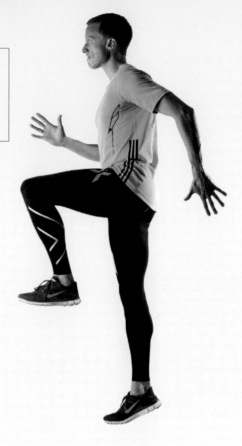

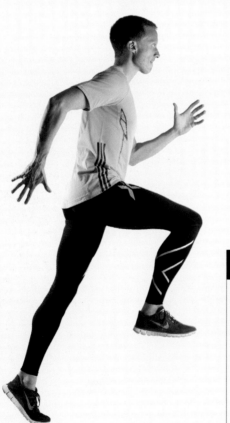

11.

Ankle walk: Start with walking in place as in exercise 10. Then, walk forward with high knees and hips in a forward position, and land with the front part of the foot under the body. You should get the sense of falling thanks to the hip position and landing under the body. Tilt the foot before it returns down and stretch in the support phase. Walk 20 meters x 2–3.

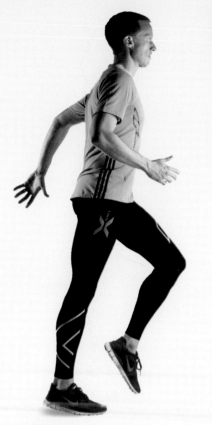

12. *Ankle run/tripping:* Push yourself forward with small and quick steps by stretching the ankle. Focus on pushing yourself forward with your hips and feet working quickly under the body. You should have ground contact throughout the exercise. Walk 20–30 meters x 2–3.

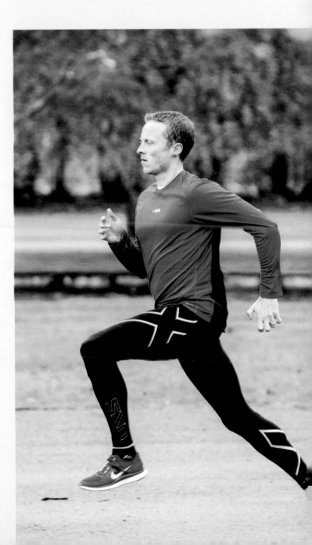

13. *Coordination run:* Run slowly with your hips tilted in the forward position with an emphasis on a quick landing on the front part of the foot. Gradually raise the tempo and keep the rapid landing. You can start with exercise 15 or 17 to find the feeling of the spring in the landing. Do 3–5 x 60–100 meters and walk back from each stretch.

IN ALL JUMP EXERCISES YOU SHOULD FOCUS ON minimizing time on the ground and maximizing the time in the air. Remember to land a little more on the whole foot (but certainly not on the heel) than when running because gravity is stronger when you jump. It's important that the load is not too large.

If you are going to be able to store and use the elastic energy, you must not collapse but must quickly push off the ground. When you do this right, the muscles are charged with elastic energy that gives you the rebound effect in the push-off. If you jump on soft ground, then you reduce the stress and risk of injury.

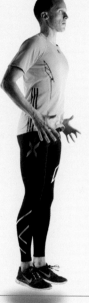

14.

Ankle jumps in place: Jump up vertically, angling your feet up in the top position. Landing on your feet, push off with the front part of the foot in a quick "radical" movement. Do 10 jumps x 2–3.

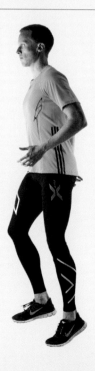

15.

Ankle bounce forward: The forward motion is roughly the same as in exercise 12, but with a more upwardly directed rebound effect that makes you lift from the ground at every step. Land with both feet at the same time but one slightly ahead of the other to move forward. For each step change front foot. Try to get the same "radical" movement as in exercise 14, meaning that you land on the whole foot and quickly push with the front of the foot. Try to learn the bouncing feeling and bring it into your running. Do 2–3 x 20–30 meters.

16.

One leg jumps: Jump right-right-left-left, with emphasis on meeting the ground with the whole foot and quickly pushing off with the front. Jump 20–30 x 3.

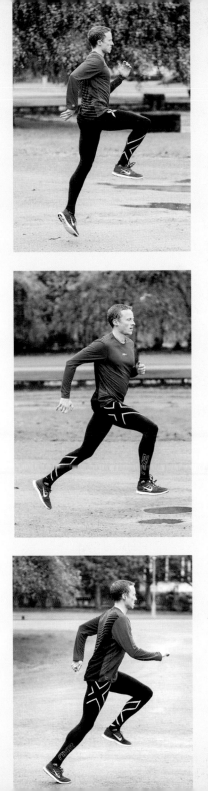

17.

Triple jump/multi step: Jump right-left-right-left, etc. It adds more stress than the other jump exercises because you land on one leg at a time. Focus on having an upright posture with the hip angled upward, so you can land underneath the body. The push-off-force will drive you forward, just like when running. If you're going to practice the elasticity in the tense muscle, then you need to be able to land with a fast and bouncy landing without collapsing. Jump 20–30 meters x 3.

18.

Single leg jump: Jump and land on the same leg with the same emphasis as in exercise 17. These are the two jump exercises that add the most stress, so ensure you are able to perform exercises 14–16 first. The first time you do them, you should practice uphill to reduce the stress. Jump 20 meters x 2 on each leg.

Get started!

Start by practicing foot strength and technique simultaneously. The foot strength program provides increased stability in the ankle. It's designed to be used regularly, you don't need to change into sportswear, and there's no need for any equipment. In technique exercises, you can practice landing with the front part of the foot under the body, which requires you to have your hip in a forward position.

Jump training provides an increased elasticity in your muscles, and is therefore both a strength and technique exercise. You get stronger ankles from jumping, which gives more rebound force in the foot landing and a longer stride.

Just remember that jumping causes more stress on the body than running, and therefore you must jump technically correctly, otherwise the effect fails, and the risk is great that you will instead hurt yourself. Start with the less demanding jump exercises and wait for 17 and 18 until you get used to jumping.

Barefoot jumping, then? Yes, it's good for your running technique, and it is also strength training for the ankles. You can practice technique exercises barefoot if you do so on a soft surface. It is, however, recommended that you wear shoes when you jump as the stress is much greater.

Remember that it's better to do fewer repetitions with proper technique than to rush through an entire program. The first few times you might just manage to do one or two exercises, but if you're careful, you will get better the more you practice.

Three technique sessions

If you don't want to put together your own program, you can do these three sessions. Be prepared to do level 1 dozens of times before you're ready to move on. If level 2 is too tough, you can either go back to level 1 and become even better there, or do the new exercises very slowly and maybe ask someone to film you.

THREE TECHNIQUE SESSIONS FOR THE FEET

LEVEL 1 – LEARN HOW TO LAND ACCURATELY

» Do strength and mobility exercises 1–9

» Do technique exercises 10–11. Be careful to have your hips in the correct position and land under the body

» Do coordination runs starting from exercise 11 and continue into faster running, remembering to land under the hip on the front part of the foot

LEVEL 2 – LEARN TO BOUNCE FROM THE GROUND

» Do strength and mobility exercises 1–9

» Continue doing exercises 10–11 to accustom yourself to landing underneath the body

» Focus on learning exercises 14–15, especially the bouncing feeling

» Do coordination runs, starting from exercises 14–15 and attempt to retain the bouncing landing

» Do test C from Chapter 10 every few weeks

LEVEL 3 – USE THE BOUNCE IN YOUR NORMAL RUNNING

» Try to retain the bouncing landing from exercises 17–18 to improve your elastic strength

» Feel that you're able to run with a fast and bouncy landing in your regular running, possibly with the help of a trigger that you have taken from any exercise

» Do test C from Chapter 10

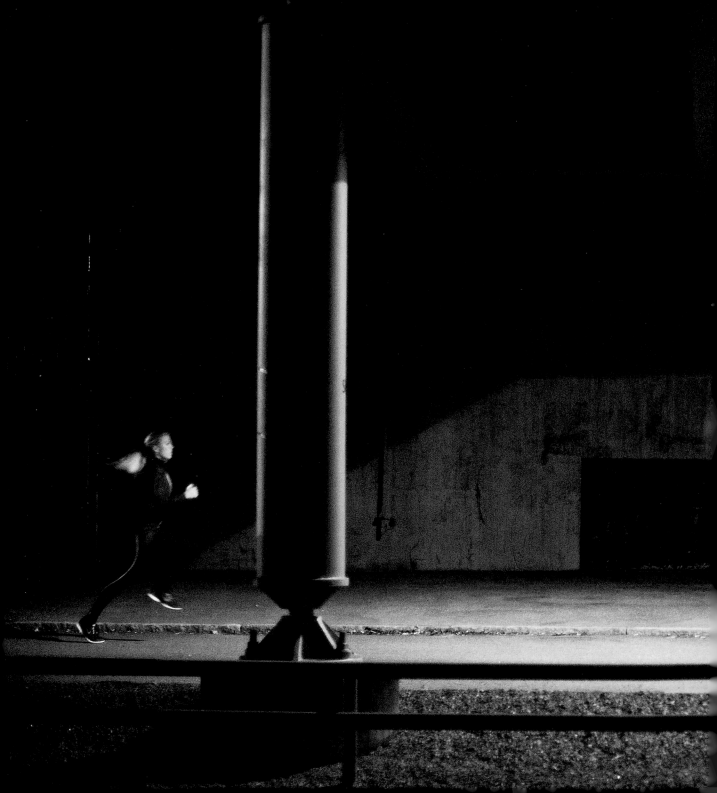

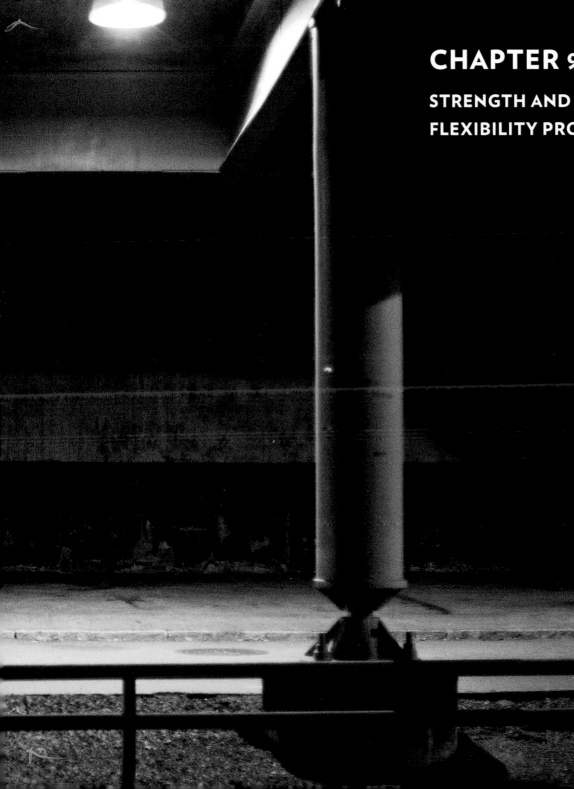

CHAPTER 9.

STRENGTH AND FLEXIBILITY PROGRAMS

9.

THE STRENGTH TRAINING PROGRAM IS DESIGNED TO BE EASY TO PERFORM. YOU DON'T NEED TO GO TO THE GYM; YOU CAN DO ALL THE EXERCISES BESIDE THE RUNNING TRACK. THE LYING DOWN EXERCISES CAN BE SWITCHED TO STANDING EXERCISES WHENEVER IT'S WET OR COLD OUTSIDE.

The program covers all the muscles you use when running. The only thing that's added is the training of the shoulders or feet for those who have chosen those technical parts.

Remember that strength-training burdens the muscles a lot more than running, and therefore you must warm up properly before the workout. A 10-minute jog and the mobility exercises on page 145–148 are normally enough. However, don't do tough cardio training before, because then the muscles are too tired for you to get any effect in their strength, and if you combine strength and technique training, you should do the technical exercises first, because they don't fatigue the muscles.

One advantage of having only your own body as the weight is that you get a broader range of motion than with machines and bars. Just like when you practice your technique, it's better to do the exercises accurately rather than training a lot or with weights that are unnecessarily heavy for long distance runners. Quality instead of quantity. Or if you like—smarter not harder.

It's enough to do exercises 1–6 once a week, while you can do exercises 7–10 twice a week with at least a couple of days in between. Choose to either do one exercise at a time or as circuit training. The advantage of the circuit is that you don't rest between the sets and will therefore also train cardio. Just remember to do the exercises accurately and not to rush them.

Remember to follow the instructions carefully for each exercise so it maximizes your strength effect and reduces the risk of injury.

1.

Heel raises with straight legs: Work with both feet up and with one foot at a time on the way down to get both concentric and eccentric strength. Stand on the steps, curb, or something similar to get a bigger range of motion (to train the outer calf muscle). Do 15 repetitions per leg x 3.

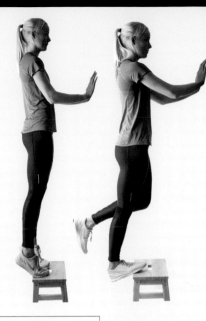

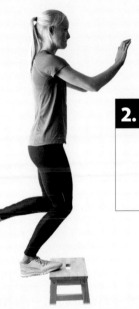

2.

Heel raises with slightly bent legs: Do the same as in the previous exercise (train the inner calf muscle). Do 15 repetitions per leg x 3.

3.

Squats: Drop the knee and hip down to a 90-degree angle and stretch upward quickly. Keep your back straight throughout the exercise and work your way down slowly so you can also train eccentrically (working the front thigh and buttocks). Do 15 repetitions x 3.

4.

Lunge walk: Be sure to have upright posture and avoid touching the ground with the knee (train the thighs front, back, and inside, and the buttocks). Walk 10 steps x 3.

5.

Reclined hip and leg lifts: Swing one leg up by pressing from the hip and the grounded leg (train the backside of the thigh, buttocks, and inner abdominals). Do 10 swings per leg x 3. If you do not want to lie on the ground, then select the reversed "plank" where you rest on your elbows with your spine facing down for about 1 minute x 3.

6.

Jackknife: Do not arch your back as it increases the stress on the back (train the hip flexors and abdominals). Repeat 15–20 x 3. If you don't want to lie on the ground, instead run with high knees uphill. Be sure to have an upright posture. Run 30 meters x 3.

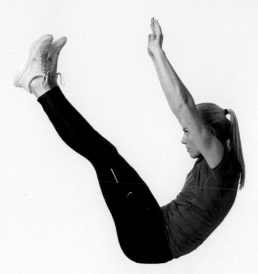

7.

Back and arm lift: Lift your head and shoulders off the ground and keep the position when you stretch your arms alternately forward and backward (train erector spinae muscles and the muscles around the shoulder blades). Do 10 x 3. If you don't want to lie on the ground, instead do circles with the arms upwards and backwards every other time. Remember to have an upright posture and make the circles as large as possible. Make 30 circles x 3.

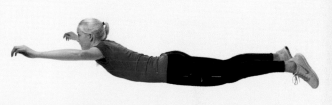

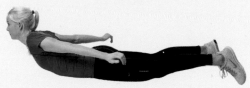

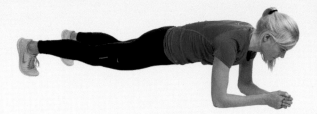

8. *"Plank"* (train inner abdominals, buttocks, and muscles in the back): Hold for about 1 minute or as long you can keep the trunk level, x 3.

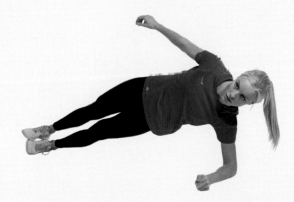

9. *"Side-plank"* (training the muscles on the side of the stomach): Do 30 seconds per side x 3.

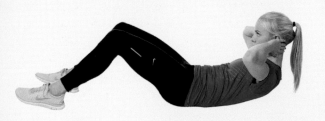

10. *Short sit-ups:* "Flatten" the lower back (train inner abdominals) 3 x max. If you don't want to lie on the ground, you can instead do a "standing plank." Tilt the pelvis by tightening the abdominals and the buttocks and stay in the upward tilted position for 30 seconds x 3.

1. *Stretch and bend:* Inhale when you stretch your arms up, exhale and lean forward without reaching all the way. Repeat 5 times.

2. *Leg swings with straight legs:* Work with a long and soft motion where you extend the grounded leg's ankle all the way. Remember to have an upright upper body and feel how the hip goes with the leg's motion. Do 10 swings back and forth with each leg.

3. *Sideways leg swings:* Keep the same emphasis as in exercise 2. Do 10 swings outward and inward on each leg.

4.

Side twist of the trunk: Lie on your back and lift your knee up toward your hand on the other side. Repeat 10 times on each side.

5.

Jog sideways with leg lift: Move sideways by lifting the trailing leg alternately in front of and behind the leading leg. Extend the movements accurately so that you rotate the hip on each step. Do 30 meters x 2.

TRY TO STRETCH after every workout to maintain muscle length. In most exercises, you can stretch out another few centimeters on each exhale and that way you can extend further out. Stretch each muscle for ten breaths or 20–30 seconds.

1.

Outer calf muscle: Keeping your back heel on the ground, press your hips forward.

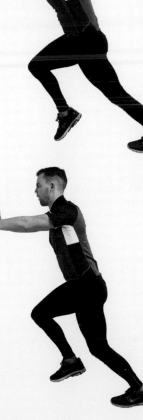

2.

Inner calf muscle: This is the same as the previous exercise but with bent knees. You should feel it a little further down towards the Achilles tendon. Press your knees forward keeping your back heel on the ground.

3. *Backside of thigh:* Arch your back and bend your front knee slightly to access the muscle. Press forward from the navel, not from the breast to gain access to the muscle and to avoid back pain.

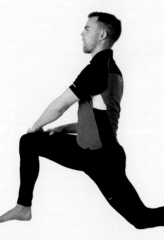

4. *The hip flexors:* Here you have to do the opposite of exercise 3 to access the muscle. Round the lower back by tilting your hips up and then push them forward.

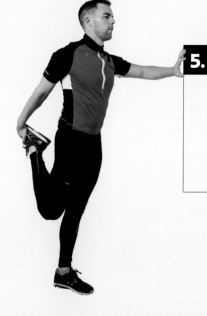

5. *Front thigh:* Try to tilt the hips while pulling your foot against the thigh without bringing your knees back. Try to lean the knee of the bent leg against a wall if it is hard to keep it in position.

6.

Outer thigh: Stand in a "skating step" so that you feel a stretch on the outside of your hips.

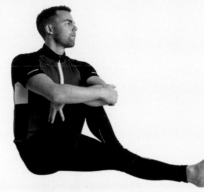

7.

Buttocks: Pull your knee inwards and push with your arms to gain access to the muscle.

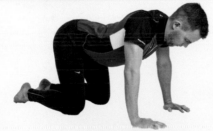

8.

Arch and round your back: Hold for 5 seconds in the extended position, repeat 2–3 times.

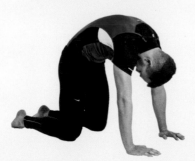

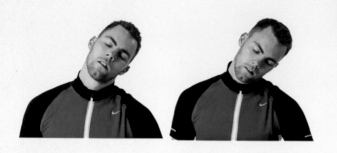

9. *Neck muscle:* Sit down. Tilt your head to the side and push the shoulder on the opposite side down to create as much distance as possible between shoulder and ear. Feel how it stretches the neck. After 20–30 seconds, tilt your head slightly forward to access the other neck muscles. Let it stretch a little further down the shoulder blades. Stay as long in this position and then switch sides.

10. *Chest muscles:* Place your elbow against a wall just above shoulder height; feel the weight of the body resting on the same side leg. Tilt the upper body forward and inward.

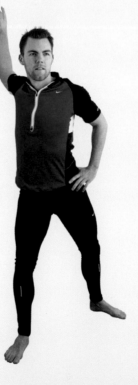

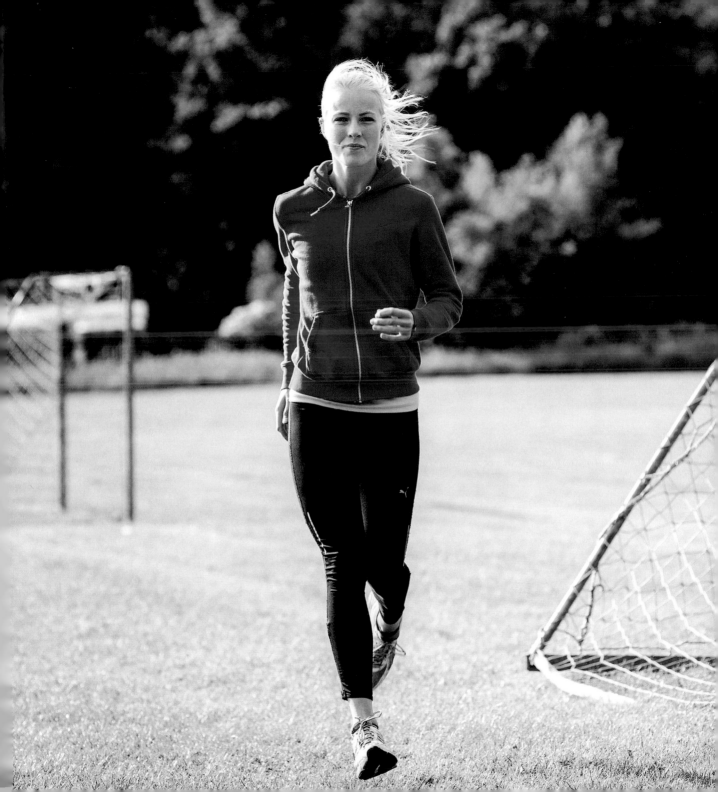

CHAPTER 10.

PUT YOUR TECHNIQUE TO THE TEST

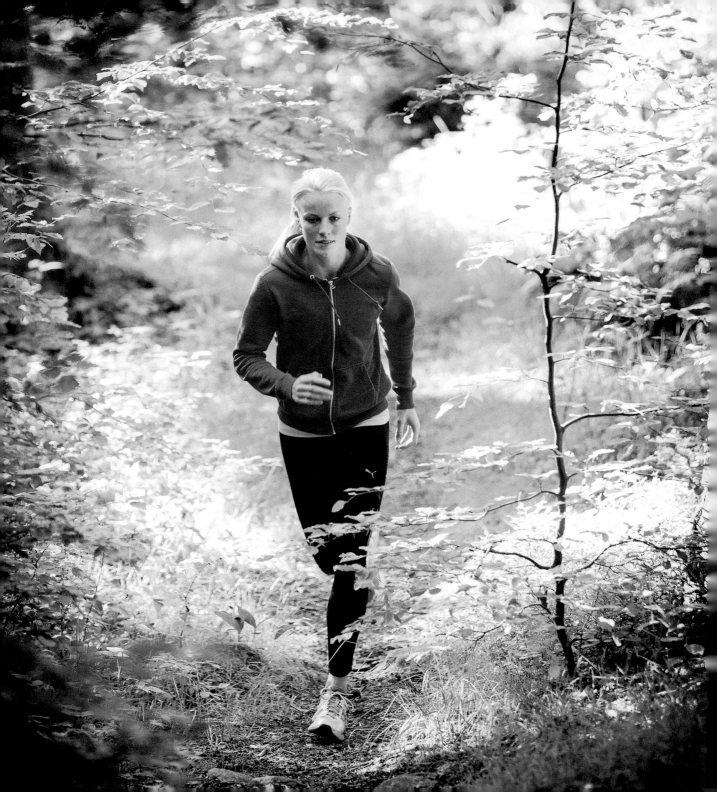

10.

USING SOME TESTS you can easily see the effect your technique training has. Tests are good for motivation and a fun break in training. Also, technical training feels more meaningful when you can improve your test results, and if the results remain unchanged after months of training, it can be a sign that you need to change something in your training.

Select one or more of the four below-mentioned tests that measure different qualities in the running stride and repeat every month. The first three set no specific requirements for training status, whereas test D requires that you have learned to jump with proper foot landing.

Remember that it is to yourself and your past performance that you should compare yourself, not to any other person. To make the tests as accurate and fair as possible, it's important that you run the same route and are as well rested each time. If you also follow the instructions carefully, it increases the quality of the test result.

A) Running economy
To use your pulse as a measurement of your running economy, you must know that it's not your fitness you are measuring. Therefore, it's important that you have about the same fitness status each time you do the test, which means your cardio training should be the same between the test sessions.

1. Run on the treadmill at a speed you can normally manage to keep to for at least 30 minutes. Measure how high your heart rate is when it stabilizes after 5–10 minutes.

2. A few weeks later, retest on a similar treadmill and at the same speed. When your running economy improves, you will have a lower heart rate than before, even though you run just as fast—you spend less energy because you have a more efficient technique.

B) Stride length
Once you get a better running technique, your stride will get longer without you thinking about it, and as a result, your running economy improves. This test measures how long your running stride is, but for it to be reliable, you should run naturally without trying to take long or short strides.

1. Measure a distance roughly 200 meters long—the important thing is that the distance is the same every time. If you cannot measure, you can run between two posts that are roughly equivalent to the distance, and that are easy to recognize so you can use the same run every time you do this test.

2. Jog up to the start and then run 200 meters pretty quickly, but relaxed. Imagine that you're going to run the pace you would have in a 500-meter sprint. Take the time and count the number of steps. If you want to increase the accuracy, then you can run in an equal way three times with at least a few minutes of rest between each race and calculate the average value for the time and number of steps. If you find it difficult to count your steps while you run, ask a friend to come and keep count. You now have the beginning value of time and stride length.

3. The most important thing when you take the test the next time is that you run at about the same speed. Try the same sprint pace as the last time, take the time and count steps, possibly as averages after three runs. The point of this test is not to see if you have be-come faster, but to find out if you're able to run the distance as quickly but with fewer steps. If you can do that without getting more tired, you will have gotten a longer running stride and a better running economy.

C) Foot landing

The most advanced way of measuring how fast you meet the ground is with the use of electronics and a contact plate. In this test you measure your landing in other ways and simultaneously train your ability to land quickly.

1. Measure a distance between two posts that are about 60 meters apart and are easy to recognize and return to the next time you do the test.

2. Jog up to the first post and run the distance quickly, yet relaxed, and with a good posture. Just as in test B above, try to run at the pace of a 500-meter sprint. For most people, this means a time between 10 and 15 seconds. Take the time and count the number of steps. If it's hard to keep count, ask a friend to stand on the sidelines and do it for you.

3. Run the 60-meter distance 3-5 more times with the objective of the same time but with about two more steps.

To do it you have to touch the ground faster and therefore the test is good training for landing. You need to have a shorter contact time by having more active feet. At the same time, the test shows how your landing has developed over time.

4. When you do the test again a few weeks later, you can compare the time and number of steps. With a better bouncing force in the ankle, you can increase the number of steps without the time being worse. Keep in mind that this is just a way to trick the body into faster foot landings—you cannot run like this in a race, where the key is to have a quick foot landing and a natural long stride.

D) Foot landing and stride length

This test measures both how fast your running stride is and the stride length. To do it, you should have trained so-called multi steps (see page 135, exercise 17).

1. Jump between two posts—the distance should be 50–60 meters apart. Count how many skips you need to do it and how long it takes. If it feels difficult, then you can make a few attempts. Note the best time and how many skips you had that time.

2. A few weeks later, retest at the same place. The goal is to reduce the number of jumps at an equally good time. To do it you need to land with even quicker feet and a more powerful push-off, which is what running is all about!

ALEXANDER R, *Energy-saving mechanisms in walking and running,* the muscle's task in running is to maximize the elastic energy, USA 1991.

ANDERSSON T, *Biomechanics and running economy*, a description of the factors that distinguish a good running economy including the conclusion that it can be achieved with technical training, USA 1996.

ARAMPATZIS A, DE MONTE G, AND KARAMANIDIS K, *Influence of the muscle-tendon unit's mechanical and morphological properties on running economy,* long distance runners with greater elasticity in their muscles have better running economy, Germany 2006.

CAVAGNA GA, SAIBENE FP AND MARGARIA R, *Mechanical work in running*, the muscles' ability to store and reuse elastic energy decreases oxygen consumption during long distance running by 25 percent, Italy 1964.

CONLEY DL, KRAHENBUHL GS, *Running economy and distance running performance of highly trained athletes,* among highly trained runners the correlation between the running ability on 10 kilometers and running economy is higher than the correlation between performance and oxygen uptake, USA 1980.

CRAIB MW and others, *The association between flexibility and running economy in sub-elite male distance runners*, increased flexibility in the hip and thigh improves running economy, USA 1996.

DAOUD AL and others, *Foot strike and injury rates in endurance runners: a retrospective study*, runners who land on the heel suffer twice as many injuries as front foot runners, and at least 74 percent of the studied runners were injured at least once in the past year, USA 2012.

DANIELS JT, *A physiologist's view of running economy*, running economy can vary by up to 30 percent among runners with the same oxygen uptake, USA 1985.

DI PRAMPERO PE and others, *Variability in energy cost of running performances in middle-distance running*, one of many studies that shows the clear correlation between running economy and the performance ability, Italy 1993.

FOSTER C, LUCIA A, *Running economy – the forgotten factor in elite performance*, research report that notes that what distinguishes East African runners from other runners is a superior running economy whereas oxygen uptake did not differ, USA-Spain 2007.

HANSON NJ, BERG K, *Oxygen Cost of Running Barefoot Vs. Running Shoed,* running barefoot reduces energy consumption by 5.7 percent; for a marathon runner who is running on 3.30, it corresponds to a decrease in time by 18 minutes, USA 2011.

KER RF, BENNETT MB, *The spring in the arch of the human foot,* when you land on the front part of the foot, the Achilles tendon and the muscles in the arch of the foot reuse 35 and 17 percent respectively of the elastic energy United Kingdom 1987.

KOMI PV, NICOL C, *Stretch-shortening cycle fatigue. Biomechanics and Biology of Movement,* Kenyan runners have better elasticity in their muscles, which explains why they recover faster and can train harder than runners from other countries, Finland 1998.

LUCIA A and others, *Physiological characteristics of the best Eritrean runners-exceptional running economy,* elite runners from Spain and Eritrea have an equally high oxygen uptake, but the Africans have almost 15 percent better running economy, which explains why they run faster, Spain, 2006.

NOAKES TD, *Implications of exercise testing for prediction of athletic performance,* for long distance runners the running economy is as important as oxygen uptake, South Africa 1988.

PAAVOLAINEN L, HAKKINEN K, *Explosive strength training improves 5-km running time by improving running economy and muscle power,* nine weeks of jump training increases the elastic muscle strength, which improves running economy by 8 percent, Finland 1999.

SJÖDIN B, SVEDENHAG J, *Applied physiology of marathon running,* running economy varies by up to 20 percent between highly trained marathon runners, Sweden 1985.

WESTON AR, MBAMBO Z AND MYBURGH KH, *Running economy of African and Caucasian distance runners,* comparison between Kenyan and European runners shows that Kenyans, due to improved running economy, can run closer to their VO_2 maximum without building up lactic acid, South Africa 2000.

WILCOX AR, BULBULIAN R, *Changes in running economy relative to VO2-max during a cross-country season,* running economy does not improve if you only train oxygen uptake, USA 1984.

ACKNOWLEDGMENTS!

A SPECIAL THANKS to the three people who have been sounding boards while working on this book:

JACOB LINDH, Sports Physiologist and Biomechanic at the Center for Health and Performance-development at the University of Gothenburg

ANDERS PALMQVIST, Development Manager for sprinter running at the Swedish Athletic Association

JOHAN WETTERGREN, Development Manager for medium and long distance running at the Swedish Athletic Association

THANKS ALSO TO those other people who contributed their knowledge:

GUSTAV FABIANSSON, Physiotherapist who, among other things, is working with the Swedish Athletic National Team

MARKUS GREUS, Physiotherapist specializing in the role of posture in sports

JOHN HELLSTROM, Research and Development Manager, the Swedish Golf Association

KLAS KULLANDER, Professor of Neuroscience, Uppsala University

ANN-CHRISTIN SOLLERHED, Senior Learning and Environment, Kristianstad University

LARS-ERIC UNESTÅHL, PhD in Applied Psychology and Mental Training

LAST BUT NOT LEAST, thank you to our models LINNEA HARRYSSON, VIBEKE BRUN, ANDREAS TOTSÅS, and JONAS HILMERSSON from Team Palmas and RICHARD MATTSSON, ALICE LUNDQVIST, and ELIN HANSTORP